Good For You

For a catalogue of related titles in our
Sexual Politics list
please write to us at an address below

Cassell
Wellington House
125 Strand
London WC2R 0BB

PO Box 605
Herndon
Virginia 20172

First published 1997

British Library Cataloguing in Publication Data
A catalogue record for this book is available from the British Library.

Library of Congress Cataloging-in-Publication Data
Wilton, Tamsin.

    Good for you: a handbook on lesbian health and wellbeing/Tamsin Wilton:
with illustrations by the author.
      p. cm.
    Includes bibliographical references and index.
    ISBN 0-304-33632-7 (pbk.)
    1. Lesbians—Health and hygiene.   2. Lesbians—Mental health.
  I. Title   RA778.2.W55 1997
  613'.04244'086643—dc21

                                                                   97-6628
                                                                  CIP

Designed and Typeset by Ben Cracknell Studios
Printed and bound in Great Britain by Redwood Books, Trowbridge, Wiltshire

Good For You

A Handbook on Lesbian Health and Wellbeing

TAMSIN WILTON

with illustrations by the author

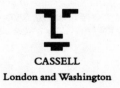

CASSELL

London and Washington

Contents

for Kim: thank you for keeping the door open

Acknowledgements

Nobody writes a book on their own, and that is particularly true in the case of a book like this one. I am very grateful to those women who took the time and trouble to read chapters that fell within their specialist area and who were so generous in making suggestions for improvements or changes. Thanks are due to Dr Rita Das, to midwives Mary Stewart and Christine Andrew, and to Hilary Lindsay for their invaluable contribution to the accuracy and helpfulness of specific chapters. Special thanks to Lesley Doyal, who read the entire manuscript (on her sickbed, no less!) and whose comments were invaluable. I have also been the lucky recipient of the kindness of other researchers who have kept me supplied with a steady stream of papers, journal articles, bibliographies and all the other fodder that is the common fare of all research but which is often so difficult to come by in the area of lesbian health. For this I am very grateful to Grindl Dockery, Clare Farquhar, Karen L. J. Hardman, Nancy Worcester, Celia Kitzinger, Hazel Platzer, Gisela Dutting, Patricia Stevens, Lesley Doyal, George Davey Smith, Jane Godfrey, Marg Hay and Sue Kippax. Thanks to you all, and I hope I can return the favour when required! I must also acknowledge LesBeWell, the lesbian health group in Birmingham, whose lesbian health research network and newsletter, *Dykenosis*, have been essential background support, and my students at the University of the West of England (UWE), many of whom have drawn my attention to things of interest. Teaching health and social care professionals is a rewarding business (on the whole!), and continually reminds me that learning is a two-way process. Special thanks to Malcolm McEachran, subject librarian at the Faculty of Health and Social Care at UWE, who broke the sacred rules of borrowing to give me extra time with my precious reference books! However, not all my encounters have been positive ones, and I have something very special to say to whoever ran off with my precious copy of *Lesbian Health Matters* and is still hanging on to it . . . GIVE IT BACK!

This book has a somewhat strange publishing history, since the proposal was initially commissioned by the Health Education Authority in England, but subsequently withdrawn when the HEA was reorganized, since it became clear that it could not be the book I wanted it to be under the new, more tightly controlled, structure. Despite this, I would never have had the idea on my own, so thanks are due to Susan Tucker, then commissioning editor at the HEA, who asked me to write the book in the first place, and to Roz Hopkins at Cassell who rescued the idea and accepted a revised version for publication.

Grateful thanks to the lesbians who shared their health care experiences with me. You have all asked to remain anonymous, so I can't thank you by name, but you know who you are, and your honesty has made a real and important contribution to this book. Finally, my own wellbeing is supported and nurtured by those people without whom I wouldn't be able to write a word: Dede Liss, Hilary Lindsay, Lesley Doyal, Stephanie Keeble, Norma Daykin and Tom Coveney.

Introduction: Why We Need a Book on Lesbian Health

When I said that I was writing a handbook on lesbian health, some people were puzzled. Non-lesbians wanted to know why such a thing was needed in the first place; surely, they protested, 'lesbian health' is the same as 'women's health'? Well, no, it isn't! There are many factors that have an impact on lesbian health and wellbeing which simply do not affect non-lesbians, and I discuss these throughout the book. There are also major flaws in most health handbooks for 'women'. On the whole, they are really health handbooks for *heterosexual* women (although they fail to acknowledge this), since they generally neglect to recognize that lesbians exist. Any lesbian who turns to such books for help and information about her health is likely to feel at best ignored and at worst hurt and infuriated. While we are all too used to feeling invisible and pushed out, this is particularly damaging when we are in need of advice about our health and wellbeing.

There are also some fairly major problems for lesbians trying to make sense of the not-so-hidden messages about how to be a good girl, which saturate so many mainstream health handbooks. Although books written from a feminist perspective may make some attempt to recognize that not all women are heterosexual, or that we do not all fall into traditional sterotypes of femininity, those written without a feminist analysis often promote sexist and damaging ideas. Take this example from women's health media guru Miriam Stoppard:

There is no doubt that many women who feel they have to adopt male standards . . . to achieve success are not only making it difficult for themselves but they may be making themselves unhappy. Such behaviour is difficult for most women because they are . . . acting unnaturally in being overly assertive.[1]

In other words, all this feminism business is bad for your health! Stoppard is also keen to promote the interests of the cosmetics industry, and advises her reader to: 'Moisturize [skin] at least twice a day . . . Wear makeup . . . blanch the skin [of your elbows] with preparations like lemon juice[2] . . . only wear rubber gloves for dirty jobs if you wear cotton gloves underneath, soaked in hand cream'.[3] This is a *health* handbook, yet Stoppard seems to see no contradiction in encouraging women to spend large amounts of time, energy (and money) on trying to conform to ideals of white heterosexual female attractiveness. All too often women's health is presented in this way, under the umbrella term 'health and beauty', powerfully reinforcing the idea that attractiveness to men is the foremost goal of a woman's existence. Such unquestioned assumptions mean that the majority of women's health guides are deeply heterosexist. This makes them inappropriate for lesbian readers but, worse still, they actively collude with the oppression of lesbians by presenting heterosexuality and its associated submissive female role as normal, natural and healthy. Such ideas are damaging to the health of lesbians.

However, lesbians have not ignored this sad state of affairs, and a small number of handbooks on lesbian health are already available. Do we really need another one? My preliminary research confirmed that many lesbians in Britain either are unaware of the existence of such books or have not found them helpful. There seems to be much dissatisfaction with the few lesbian health books that already exist, either because they are written exclusively for a North American readership or because of their political perspective (or both). It is not always possible to get hold of them unless you have access to a lesbian and gay or women's bookshop, and these tend to be found only in larger cities. Your local mainstream bookshop is unlikely to stock them, especially since existing lesbian health handbooks have been brought out by small, independent publishing houses who often lack access to the major book distributors. The costs of importing books in small numbers means that a book published by a small press in the USA will not be easily available in Britain, and is likely to be expensive. As far as I know, this is the first lesbian health handbook to be published by a large mainstream publishing house; as such it should be easily available to lesbians throughout the English-speaking world. I owe a great debt to the work done by these independent lesbian and feminist publishers; their books are invaluable to lesbians everywhere, they have been the trailblazers in this field and they continue to set the agenda for lesbian publishing. However, it is not surprising that their books can be somewhat inward-looking, addressing the small communities which produced them, and uncritically reflecting the values of those communities.

Because there is no straightforward guide to lesbian health freely available to lesbians in Britain, this one is written from a British perspective and is primarily addressed to British lesbian readers, although I have included material which is specifically relevant to lesbians in the United States, Canada and other countries where appropriate. It is a book about and for lesbians, but I hope that it will also be read by health professionals who want to find out how best to provide effective services to their lesbian patients and clients, since there is precious little else available on this subject.

I have also tried to make sure that this handbook is useful to as many different 'kinds' of lesbian as possible. Of course I have my own perspective and beliefs, but I do not think that it is my business to foist them on women who are looking for information and advice on health. Health, perhaps especially lesbian health, is an unavoidably political issue and I have discussed it as such. However, it is not helpful to individual lesbians, or to lesbian communities, to use words like 'unhealthy' to stigmatize behaviours (such as consensual sadomasochism or having sex with men) which some lesbians may disapprove of. Your discomfort does not give you the right to label other lesbians 'sick' or 'unhealthy'. These tactics have long been used against us, and it is in nobody's interests if the oppressed begin to mimic the strategies of the oppressor.

The business of writing this book brought me face to face with some of the ways in which our lives as lesbians can put stress on our health and wellbeing. It was turned down by a major feminist publisher on the grounds that there wasn't enough demand – an excuse which ironically echoes the reasons mainstream institutions generally give for refusing to take lesbians into consideration. As lesbians, we are used to having our lives and needs dismissed as unimportant or irrelevant, and dealing with this kind of disrespect on a daily basis takes its toll on our physical and emotional wellbeing. Then there are the practicalities of finding the time to research and write a book like this. As a single parent I have to generate a regular income; I am lucky enough to be able to do this by working at a job I love, but it still means that my 'lesbian work', such as writing this book, has to be done in my own time on top of my other (full-time) job and running my home. After a hard day preparing and giving lectures, guiding students through various crises, working up research funding bids and attending meetings, committees and seminars I would stagger home, feed self, son and cats and sit down at the word processor or drawing board. My idea of a fun day off now means having the time to wash some clothes and vacuum a room or two without having to digest a research paper on bacterial vaginosis or multi-infarct dementia. Guess what? Working like that is stressful, exhausting and bad for you! By the end of the book repetitive strain injury had extended from my hands to my elbows and shoulders, the all-too-familiar signs of stress and exhaustion were dominating my daily life, and my social life had dwindled to a staunch handful of loved and loyal friends, leavened with the uplifting but sporadic whirlwind presence of my teenage son and the variously dependable affections of five cats. Without my daily, obsessively ritualized, cup of coffee, this book would never have been written. So there is really no way I could lecture you, gentle reader, on the evils of your own chosen drugs of solace.

I should also mention that I have been inspired by the enthusiastic support given to this project by so many lesbians working in the field of health. Time after time my polite letters asking for information met with excited replies and bundles of useful material. It has been a very special experience to feel nourished and encouraged by this dedicated network of lesbian energy from the USA to the Netherlands, to South Africa, to Australia, to Ireland. I hope that this book may be, among other things, a way into some of that energy for lesbians who need it.

How to use this book

Depending on what you want to get out of it, you can use this book in two ways. If you want to become better informed about lesbian health generally, it has been designed to be reader-friendly, and the chapters do follow a sequence which makes some sort of sense. So feel free to read it from cover to cover. However, many of us reach for a health handbook when we need advice about something specific. Maybe you suspect that you are approaching menopause, and you want to check out ways in which this might be different for lesbians. Or perhaps you are wondering whether it is time to have the baby you have always wanted, and you would appreciate a little basic advice and information. In which case, the chapters have been written to act as informative introductions to specific health concerns. Obviously, a book of this size cannot contain definitive advice on every health issue faced by every lesbian. If it did, you would have to spend six months at the gym to be able to lift it (and a year to be able to read it in bed). So each chapter concludes with a section listing further reading and the general chapters also include other resources, such as groups, helplines and newsletters, which you may find helpful. These sections are quite short, but each resource listed will lead you in turn to many others.

This book is *not* intended to replace a doctor's advice, and is not a manual of self-treatment. It is important to seek properly qualified advice if you suspect that something is wrong, and you should not assume that your own interpretation of your experiences is necessarily correct. On the other hand, nor is it necessarily wrong! For example, many of the early signs of menopause mimic warning signs of diabetes, and this on its own means that it is well worth while paying a visit to a doctor to check out what is going on. I am a great believer in making use of whatever sources of help, advice and treatment are available to you, and that includes scientific medicine, homoeopathy, acupuncture, herbalism, support groups or whatever. However, all of these vary enormously in the extent to which they are lesbian-friendly, or in their degree of ignorance about lesbian needs and concerns. This book is intended to be one of those sources of help and advice, and it is a particularly lesbian-friendly one, with an emphasis on lesbian needs and concerns.

I was able to talk to a small number of lesbians about their experiences with health and the health care system. They all spoke to me on condition that they remained anonymous, since the risks involved in being identified as a lesbian were too great for any of them to take that risk. That in itself is a powerful indicator of the stresses which may impact on our health! I have also drawn on some already published accounts of individuals' experiences; not all of these are from lesbians (although the great majority are), and no assumptions about anyone's sexuality should be drawn from the fact that their words are used in this way.

Being a lesbian is undoubtedly health-promoting: exciting, rewarding, nourishing and deeply pleasurable. But surviving as a lesbian in a society rotten with homophobia, sexism, racism, disability oppression, ageism, anti-semitism and all the other horrors demands extraordinary courage, strength and belief in oneself. Yet we all do it. Each and every day of our lives. Which makes us a very wonderful people, and makes me proud to call myself a lesbian. I hope this book will make things a little easier.

1 What's So Special About Lesbians?

The very idea of lesbian health seems peculiar to some people. After all, our bodies are not noticeably different from those of non-lesbian women; contrary to superstition and some 'medical' folklore we don't have horns or abnormal genitals,[1] and there are no special lesbian diseases. What is more, we have not yet entirely won our fight against the idea that lesbianism is in itself some kind of disease, sickness, disability or (at best) a symptom of underlying pathology. Not only does it seem unnecessary to consider lesbian health at all, but it could be argued that writing about lesbians as a distinct group with specific health needs comes a bit too close to some of the most oppressive and offensive ideas that the medical profession has disseminated about us as 'sick' people. So, what's so special about lesbian health?

Lesbian health is special on two counts. First, research indicates that there are health consequences linked to having sex with women, not having sex with men and being less likely to become pregnant and give birth. These consequences are, in fact, more likely to be beneficial rather than a risk to women's health, although there do seem to be some potential health risks associated with being lesbian. This knowledge is clearly extremely significant for lesbians. Not only is it very useful to be informed about potential health risks in order to take what steps we may to safeguard our own health, but also it is very important that lesbians are aware of the many ways in which being lesbian is actively health-promoting. Against a cultural backdrop of profound hostility against lesbians, such information can be strengthening and affirming.

The second concern of this book is the relationship between our health and society. For, while being a lesbian may be good for you, living in a society which hates lesbians is most assuredly bad for you. In this, lesbians are not unique. Health is a complex issue, and if health research has taught us anything over the course of the twentieth century it is that you cannot understand health or illness if you think in purely biological or medical terms. The key question in health is why, when exposed to the same disease-causing organisms or potentially damaging situations, some people become ill and others do not. The answer lies in understanding what makes us *vulnerable* to ill health, and this vulnerability is intimately linked to our position in society. Sociologists have known for a long time that people in the lower social classes suffer more acute illnesses, accidental injuries and chronic sickness than those in higher social classes, that they die at an earlier age and that their children are more likely to die around birth or during infancy.[2] The dramatic improvements in the health of populations living in the wealthy industrialized nations this century are due not to advances in medical knowledge such as vaccination or new drugs but to improved living conditions, proper sanitation and better food, all of which are more readily available to privileged groups.

It is not just social class which has such a dramatic impact on health and life chances, and 'privilege' means more than just having lots of money. Researchers have found that gender and ethnicity – or, rather, sexism and racism – have a clear influence on health. Similar research into lesbian and gay health is relatively new, but already there are findings which suggest quite clearly that the stigmatized social position of lesbians and gay men may be very damaging to our physical and emotional health and wellbeing. Once you begin to look at lesbians in the context of the societies in which we have to live, it becomes all too clear that, for many women, living as a lesbian is a constant struggle.

Moreover, lesbians are never 'just' lesbians. Women are more likely than men to be living in poverty, and this is as true of lesbians as it is of non-lesbian women.[3] Working-class lesbians will suffer the disadvantages of their socio-economic status. Lesbians who are Jewish or black, from minority communities or of mixed race will be affected by racism and anti-semitism. Lesbians have only one thing in common, our choice to act on our loves and desires for women. Set that aside and 'lesbians' are as disparate a group of women as you could hope to find, including members of all other oppressed groups. Even the consequences of our sexuality are shaped by our differences. As a white, relatively able-bodied teacher in a university I get punished all the time for being a lesbian, but the ways in which I am punished are not the same as the ways in which society punishes lesbians who are black, or severely impaired, or homeless, or addicted to street drugs, or who turn tricks or work in low-paid, low-status jobs. Sexism, classism, racism and homophobia all intersect in the lives of all of us, and all have health consequences. This book looks at the health consequences of lesbian oppression and suggests ways in which they may be minimized.

The trouble with doctors: lesbians and the medical profession

Health care professionals work with us when we are at our most vulnerable. Deciding to seek medical attention almost always means that you are feeling ill and/or worried and any kind of serious or prolonged illness is frightening. We expect those who choose to work in health care to be able to provide good and appropriate care, and to have the skills needed to communicate effectively with us and to reassure us when neccessary. Such skills are perhaps rarer than we may hope in any case, but for lesbian patients they are still more uncommon. Unfortunately, few non-lesbian health care workers have the information and skills they need to provide effective care to lesbians; moreover, they are all too often ignorant and prejudiced.[4] But the ignorance and homophobia of individuals in the health care workforce is not the only problem which confronts lesbians who seek good and effective care. Medical science itself has a deeply troubling history with regard to lesbianism; a brief look at that history makes it all too clear just how deeply implicated medicine has been in maintaining the homophobic prejudices of society as a whole.

From the start, medical science has regarded lesbianism as a problem to be solved. Indeed it is only relatively recently that *some* scientists in *some* cultures have stopped insisting that love and sexual desire between women is a pathological condition to be cured. Throughout human history there have been attempts to 'explain' same-sex desire, and such explanations have inevitably been couched in the intellectual framework which was available at the time. At those times in European history when the Christian religion was dominant, for example, sexual activity between two men or two women was seen as a sin. Engaging in such acts generally didn't mean you were any special kind of person, just someone who had fallen into temptation. However, scientific explanations have generally tended to differ from these early religious explanations by seeking a cause for such behaviour in the body or personality of the person concerned, thus inevitably giving rise to the idea that experiencing sexual desire for a member of your own sex indicated that you were somehow intrinsically different from 'normal' people.

The history of these explanations is a curious one, which throws light on the troubled relationship between the group of people we now think of as lesbian or gay, and the scientists who demonstrate such eagerness to classify us. From the Greece of Plato to early medieval Europe, homosexuality was seen as a failure of *gender*, and explanations of homosexuality were linked to whatever explanation of gender was popular among writers of the time. This is probably the gravest mistake which heterosexual thinkers have made in trying to understand same-sex love and desire, but it continues to shape scientific attempts to explain lesbianism right up to the present moment.[5]

Most 'modern' scientific theories are trapped in the belief that lesbianism is an inherent property of certain kinds of body. In the 1950s it was fairly commonly believed that lesbians could be distinguished from heterosexual women by their genitals. In 1950 the Committee for the Study of Sex Variants commissioned a study by one George W. Henry MD into the shape and behaviour of the genitals (and even the nipples!) of lesbians and gay men. Henry published a report containing detailed drawings of such gems as 'typical sex variant vulva', 'short, broad vulva, homosexual' and 'composite drawing of male and female sex variant pelves [pelvises]', all in the interests of proving that lesbianism was caused by, or could be diagnosed by, specific characteristics of the body, especially the genitals.[6] When you think about it, this is absurd. Trying to prove that women who prefer sex with other women have peculiarly shaped vaginas makes as much sense as trying to prove that vegetarians have peculiarly shaped mouths! Unfortunately, being silly has never stopped medical research. One medical doctor, Frank Caprio, stated that some lesbians have 'an unusually elongated clitoris' and that in some cases these were as much as six centimetres long, while David Reuben (another doctor) insisted that some lesbians possess a clitoris 'as much as two or more inches in length when erect', and that 'lesbians with this anatomical quirk are very much in demand'.[7] Clearly such bizarre ideas spring from the assumption that lesbians are in some way 'like' men, and so must have some kind of penis in order to have sex with women. In similar vein other researchers investigated homosexual muscle strength (by measuring hand grip), ability to whistle (an obvious sign of masculinity!) and body build, concluding that lesbians 'look more solid' than non-lesbian women, have 'bigger busts and waists', and 'mostly look older than their age'.[8]

Such naive and unsophisticated experiments became obsolete as medical technology developed, enabling researchers to focus on hormones, brain structure and (eventually) DNA in the continuing attempt to discover something peculiar about the homosexual body. Not surprisingly, most of these experiments have focused on gay men; there are few which include lesbians. Nevertheless, the fact that so much time, effort and money continues to be directed to this project – at a time when biomedical research has many more pressing problems to solve and in the teeth of increasing cuts in research funding – has important implications for lesbians' health and wellbeing.

When the so-called 'discovery' of the 'gay gene' was under discussion, many gay men and some lesbians were enthusiastic about the idea that homosexuality might be discovered to be biologically determined. Their argument went along the lines of 'Since it is in our genes, we can't help it and it is unjust to discriminate against us'. This has always struck me as a profoundly ignorant and naive perspective. After all, women can't help being born women, and black people can't help being born black. Yet this has never stopped sexism or racism. It is important for all of us to understand the implications of these attempts to 'fix' homosexuality in the body.

First, the drive to find a 'gay gene' is based on the assumption that, for a man to love and desire another man or for a woman to love and desire another woman, *something must have gone wrong with their bodies*. In other words, homosexuality is presented as pathological, a breakdown, developmental failure or disease of the otherwise 'normal' body. Second, every effort to find the cause, or evidence, of homosexuality in the body – whether is it to do with genital configuration, hormonal abnormality, genetic malformation or neurological malfunction – is linked to the suggestion that, once found and understood, *something can be done about it*. Whether this involves hormonal treatment (as has been tried with convicted 'sex offenders', most notoriously during experiments on gay prisoners in the Nazi death camps), surgical gender 'reassignment' (as with so-called sex-change surgery) or simply aborting 'gay' foetuses, the belief behind all this research is that homosexuality should and can be eradicated. This makes it difficult for lesbians and gay men to trust doctors, and difficult for the medical profession to respond appropriately to the needs of its lesbian and gay clients. In addition, decades of feminist research have shown that many doctors and other health care professionals are profoundly sexist, holding unhelpful prejudices and beliefs about women which can have a very direct influence on the care we receive. Women who are ill are all too often seen as hypochondriacal, attention-seeking or neurotic. Lesbian therapist Ricky Boden concludes that 'a woman's physical symptoms and emotional reactions to symptomatology are more likely to be ignored, labeled psychogenic ["all in the mind"] or minimized'.[9] So lesbians, being both homosexual *and* female, have a doubly difficult relationship with the medical profession.

With friends like these?
The women's health movement

The women's health movement has been one of the most successful consequences of the revitalized women's movement which emerged in Europe, Australia and the United States in the 1960s and 1970s. Feminist health activists have been successful in demonstrating the sexism of the medical establishment, the widespread mistreatment of women seeking health care, and the extent to which medical science defined 'healthy' 'normal' femininity in ways that colluded with women's oppression and secondary social status. Around the world, from the urban jungles of New York or Glasgow to thousands of small, traditional rural communities, the health care available to women has changed as a result of decades of feminist activism. Yet, in spite of all this activity, the health care needs of lesbians remained invisible until very recently.

The relationship between the women's movement and lesbians has not been an easy one, and the failure of feminist health activists to address lesbian health is not surprising in the light of a general failure within feminism to take lesbian issues on board. While there is not enough space here to discuss the history of conflict between lesbians and feminists,[10] it is important to recognize that the women's health movement has been almost as saturated with homophobia, with heterosexist assumptions and with open hostility towards lesbians as mainstream society. The consequences of this can be seen in the resources and services which grew out of feminist health activism.

A quick look at some of the books which feminist authors have written on women's health issues exposes a widespread failure to address the needs of lesbians. Bearing in mind that lesbian activists have been extremely vocal in drawing attention to this neglected issue throughout the 1980s and 1990s, it might be expected that any book on women's health written from a feminist perspective in the 1990s would – at the very least – deal adequately with lesbian concerns. Yet a glance at four fairly typical books (*Women's Health Guide* by Ann Furedi and Mary Tidyman, *Women and Disability: The Experience of Physical Disability Among Women* by Susan Lonsdale, *Women, Health and Medicine* by Agnes Miles, and Peggy Foster's *Women and the Health Care Industry: An Unhealthy Relationship?*) quickly reveals that the word 'women', when used by non-lesbian feminist writers, generally means 'heterosexual women'. The reader should reasonably expect that a health care handbook, an account of the experiences of disabled women, a feminist exploration of women's health and a critical account of women's relationship with the health care industry would all have plenty to say about lesbians; yet, between them, these four books contain *twenty-nine lines* about lesbians. Susan Lonsdale recognizes that disabled women are assumed to be heterosexual (although she herself continually makes the same assumption throughout the rest of her book). Agnes Miles does not recognize that lesbians exist (despite writing about topics such as doctor/patient interactions or substance abuse, where lesbian issues are known to be significant). Peggy Foster mentions the fact that lesbians have restricted access to alternative insemination, and thinks it is a pity that lesbians are being encouraged to use dental dams for safer sex (while ignoring lesbians in the context of mental health, cancer, health promotion, maternity care and the menopause). And Furedi and Tidyman offer the brusque information 'Lesbian: where women are attracted to other women', and comment that 'Lesbians do not just identify themselves as lesbians when they are having sex with another woman; their sexual preferences shape the rest of their lives too.' For these to be the *only* references made to lesbians in these recently published books on women's health is unacceptable and offensive.

If non-lesbian feminists have relegated lesbian health to obscurity, feminist lesbians have all too often approached the question of lesbian health from a judgemental and moralistic perspective, or with narrow political correctness. This means that, of the few resources available to lesbians who are concerned about their health, most address themselves to the chosen few, a handful of politically (and chemically) pure women who advocate a specific brand of lesbian feminism. Distressingly typical is Cuca Hepburn and Bonnie Gutierrez's (1994) book, *Alive and Well: A Lesbian Health Guide*, which promotes a twelve-step addiction model as unproblematic, and has nine *pages* of judgemental abuse against lesbian sadomasochists, including such gems as this:

Just as Lesbian communities support recovering alcoholics with substance-free events, we can support recovering sadomasochists by helping them channel their erotic impulses positively. They can be helped to see all the choices available to them sexually.[11]

Such patronizing (and ignorant) moralism is simply inappropriate in the pages of a lesbian health handbook, where lesbians who enjoy sadomasochism should be entitled to expect information about sexual health in the context of S/M. It is hard to believe that the authors, who are well aware of the damage done to lesbian self-esteem by the negative views of mainstream society, believe that promoting this kind of negative attitude to lesbians with specific sexual desires is good for their health and wellbeing!

This moralism sometimes seems to take the form of internalized guilt and homophobia. It is almost as if, having grown up in a climate of hostility towards lesbians, in societies that insisted that lesbianism was a sickness and lesbian sex is unnatural, we feel obliged to regurgitate these messages ourselves. For example, in a brief chapter outlining lesbian health needs, Karen Kerner speculates that penetration may be dangerous to lesbian health:

Cervical cancer is usually asymptomatic . . . In addition, no one knows the effects on the cervix of constant battering by penetrating sex toys and fists. It may be that . . . repeated minor trauma to the cervix predisposes lesbians to inflammation, infections and cancer.[12]

No right-wing moral majority zealot could do better than this! With no evidence whatsoever, Kerner seems to feel it is necessary to scare lesbians off penetrative sex by threatening them with cervical cancer. A moment of thoughtful contemplation (or wider research among lesbians) would surely have prevented this hysterical scare-mongering: 'battering' of the cervix is painful and unlikely to be the 'constant' practice of anyone; in any case 'battering' is not an accurate description either of fisting or of how you generally use sex toys; if either fisting or dildos really *did* lead to infections, we would have noticed by now, and *no link whatsoever* has ever been demonstrated between minor trauma to the cervix and cancer. Doctors writing about the sexual health of heterosexual women do not warn them about the 'constant battering' of the cervix by penises during heterosex; why does a lesbian doctor seem so eager to suggest that lesbian sexual activity is brutal and harmful?

The problem with much health advice to lesbians is that it is potentially damaging to the health of those readers whose behaviour does not conform to the moral standards of the author. If you enjoy S/M, Hepburn and Gutierrez's desire to heal you won't do much for your self-esteem; if you like penetration, Kerner's dire warnings about cancer are not going to reduce your anxiety levels, and the goddess

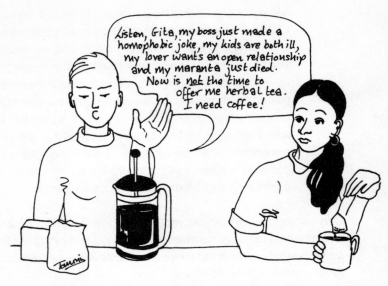

help you if you indulge in horrific practices like drinking coffee or milk.[13] Of course it is important to have as much information as possible about the potentially harmful effects of pleasurable activities and, of course, every lesbian has the absolute right to refuse to indulge in coffee, S/M, penetration or anything else if she has reason to believe that it is not good for her. But this does not give anyone the right to try to enforce their own moral agenda by using death and disease as threats. These have been the familiar tactics of authoritarian moralists ever since scare campaigns warned a terrified population that masturbation would lead to insanity, dribbling, blindness and hairy palms.[14] It is difficult enough for lesbians to maintain our wellbeing in a hostile society, without having to combat hostility within our own communities. Lesbians have the right to adequate information about health whatever choices we make in our lives and relationships.

Living in a ghetto?
Some problems with lesbian culture

The social aspects of lesbian life are more likely to damage our health than the physical activities of having sex with each other. Being a lesbian means choosing to call yourself by a name which is widely mocked, hated and feared. It means having to invest energy every day of our lives in protecting our emotional, psychological and physical wellbeing in a generally hostile context. We all live our lives in the certain knowledge that there are many people out there who wish us dead because we love and desire each other and choose to act on that love and desire. The stresses that trouble other people – poverty, job insecurity, parenting and relationship problems, housing, etc. – are all associated with additional problems for us. Living in the midst of all this stress it is a source of wonder and amazement that most of us manage to build fulfilling, creative, whole and mostly happy lives. By any standards, we are extraordinary people!

Our communities too, of course, develop and grow in the belly of the beast, in the front line of the war against homophobia. They can offer support, sanctuary, challenge and a family. Not surprisingly, they can also promote values which are warped by the constant battle against a hostile mainstream. Sometimes such community values, the values of the front line, are potentially damaging to our health. This is often called internalized homophobia, but much of what we do to one another in the name of the lesbian nation, or of sisterhood or of the feminist revolution, does not need such a sophisticated psychological description. The idea of internalized homophobia implies that deep down within each of us lurks the belief that the hatred of lesbians which our society promotes is well founded, and that the dreadful stereotypes about lesbians which we have all been exposed to (that we are all fat, ugly, infantile creatures who cannot cope with being female, cannot get a man or really want to *be* men) are true.

There is no doubt that internalizing such beliefs is probably an inevitable part of growing up in cultures where lesbians are hated and it is only too likely that each of us struggles with such beliefs in different ways. However, you don't need internalized homophobia in order to treat other lesbians badly, to bully them, trash them, lay down the law about how they should behave or set up hopelessly unreachable goals for all true lesbians to meet. You just need to be scared. Authoritarian behaviour is almost always a response to being scared, and any lesbian who trashes S/M dykes or mocks vanilla dykes, who decries non-vegetarian lesbians, drug-using lesbians or lesbians who have sex with men, or who declares that lesbians who like penetration are, in Julia Penelope's infamous jibe, 'lesbians from the waist down', is probably very scared. Unfortunately, being scared is a realistic and rational response to being hated by the most powerful groups in society, and there is a lot of fear in most lesbian communities, all too often masquerading as political commitment. This is not to decry political commitment, or to suggest that we replace political analysis with personal growth; I think we need both, and somehow we have to find a way of integrating them.

Of power and powerlessness

At the root of lesbian oppression is the question of power. Often we talk and write about power as if we all knew what it meant, but if you spend a few minutes trying to define it you will soon realize that it is very difficult to get a handle on. The kind of power which is involved when you lose your job for coming out at work is not the same as the power of love, or the power which fuels you to overcome all obstacles and achieve a longed-for goal. The sort of power which lesbians are routinely deprived of in mainstream Western societies is the power to make our own choices. Because women are poorer than men, because the labour market is biased in favour of men, because governments are controlled by men, the professions are run by men and the education system is dominated by men, men get to take control – although often at one remove – of women's choices. Because homophobia is such a powerful (and respectable) element of Western cultures, there are additional restrictions on the choices and opportunities available to lesbians. We are used to having very little power in our lives.

Unfortunately, this means that there is often a very confused idea of power sloshing round in many lesbian (and, indeed, feminist) circles. One good example is the celebratory approach of some fat liberationists, who insist that being fat is *the same as* being powerful. Typical of this approach is one fat lesbian who comments:

I really believe that fat is power. Personally, I think that's why men have been on our asses to get smaller, because we are powerful. I think that I'm a very powerful person. The larger I am, the more powerful I become.[15]

Although it may be important for her self-esteem for this woman to experience her fat as power, this does not mean that the lesbian community should be content with the idea that power equals size. There is no doubt that the cultural pressure on women (and increasingly men) to be slim is damaging to the health and self-esteem of millions and puts lorry-loads of money in the pockets of the slimming industry. But how politically useful is it if the only kind of power we can imagine is the power to take up more space? Are we really naive enough to believe that men's power will crumble if we all get fatter? Moreover, it is not true that all the risks of being fat are simply invented by the diet industry in order to get their hands on our money. Nor is being fat in any sense 'natural', except in (very rare) cases of metabolic disorder. We become fat by eating more food than our bodies require – often by being fed too much during childhood, when the process is out of our control, or in response to emotional neglect or distress. You do not see many fat people in poor communities in the Third World. You see a lot of fat people in the United States, the richest country in the world, which consumes an obscene proportion of the world's resources. But it is *not* the rich and powerful people in the USA who are fat. Obesity is overwhelmingly found among the poorest and most disenfranchized groups in American society. This suggests that fat, far from being any form of power, is some kind of compensation for powerlessness.

None of this is to suggest that lesbian communities should not be challenging fat oppression, or that any lesbian should be discriminated against on grounds of weight. But we need to think very carefully about the implications of celebrating fat as power. Many of us may use food (rather than alcohol, street drugs, obsessive exercise, self-injury or many other such strategies) as a way of dealing with the consequences of abuse and/or powerlessness. If we fail to recognize this we collude with the oppression of fat lesbians. Moreover, the politics of food is an international question, not just a local one, and we need to remain alert to how complex the whole question of fat is, and not to replace hard thinking with simplistic generalizations. To insist that fat is power does a grave disservice both to fat women, many of whom have very little power in their lives, and to the peoples of poor nations whose inadequate diet is a direct consequence of the greed of the First World. It also hinders our shared struggle to transform the inequalities of power which constrain our lives, by reducing the question of power to one of body-image. And power is central to the whole question of lesbian health.

Hopeful signs?

The belief system of Western scientific medicine is problematic for lesbians. Moreover, some members of the scientific medical community continue to participate in research motivated by a desire to eradicate homosexual desires and behaviours. But all is not doom and despair. There is a groundswell of activity on the part of lesbian researchers, health care workers, teachers and writers, which is effectively putting lesbian health issues on the agenda in many countries in the West. Change, as ever, is slow in coming, but quite extraordinary changes have happened already and things are improving on an almost daily basis, thanks to the individual energy and commitment of many lesbians. It is possible to detect a two-pronged approach: lesbians have been involved in developing alternatives to establishment health care and, more recently, in working to change the health care establishment itself.

The history of community-based health care is as old as the idea of a lesbian community, and owes much to the women's health movement. Since the 1970s, women's health groups and lesbian and gay community groups have set up well woman clinics, support groups, helplines, advice centres, mental health projects, drug and alcohol projects and many other front-line services for lesbians in need of health care services or advice. This voluntary sector activity has been given new impetus by the gay community response to HIV/AIDS, although many lesbians point out that gay men are not known for their energetic support of lesbian health issues in the way that lesbians have supported gay men in the context of AIDS.

It is probably true that the history of community activism on health gave lesbian health care workers the confidence and the information necessary to start building a foundation for identifying and meeting the needs of lesbians within the formal health care system. It is a foundation built in the teeth of neglect and without the resources which most health care workers would consider necessary for such an enterprise. Those holding the purse strings have generally refused to even consider funding the kind of research which is needed. Before health care system managers and policy-makers spend money on providing services for lesbians they have to be convinced that such services are necessary and cost-effective. Convincing them demands high-quality research. You have to prove to their satisfaction that, first, there are enough lesbians to make it worthwhile providing any services at all, second, that lesbians have needs which are not met by existing services and, third, that there is clearly demonstrable benefit (increasingly this is understood as *economic* benefit) in offering services to lesbians. Given that it is notoriously difficult to do research among lesbians (how do you know they are all lesbians? what definition of lesbian are you going to use? how do you get women to tell you what their sexual orientation is? why should lesbians trust a researcher anyway? how are you going to find a sufficiently large sample . . . etc. etc.), getting hold of enough data to convince funding bodies to pay for the research in the first place is a massive obstacle. *Then* you have to carry out the research, present your findings to the satisfaction of whoever funded it and somehow find a way of making sure that your findings have some sort of practical influence on those powerful enough to change policies.

It all sounds very daunting and, as anyone who has ever tried to get lesbian health research funded will tell you, it is a frustrating and exhausting business. Yet, despite all the obstacles, there is now a rapidly growing interest in lesbian health in many sectors of the health care establishment. Although the training given to doctors, nurses and the other professions allied to medicine (physiotherapists, midwives, radiographers, etc.) still makes little or no mention of lesbians, demand is growing for this to change. In Britain the Royal College of Nursing has supported a working party on lesbian and gay health for some years, and its work has resulted in the Royal College issuing a formal Statement on the health care of this group, as well as the publication of many positive articles in the nursing press. In the early 1990s Dr Jane Kavanagh set up specialist lesbian sexual health clinics – the Audre Lorde and Sandra Bernhardt – in two major London hospitals, whose success has prompted the establishment of similar clinics in Oxford, Glasgow and other British cities. Perhaps most important of all are the efforts to co-ordinate research in this field, to share findings and prevent lesbians having to invent the wheel on a daily basis. For example, in Britain the Birmingham group LesBeWell produces a regular health newsletter for lesbians, *Dykenosis*, as well as co-ordinating a research network for lesbian health, while in the USA the National Lesbian and Gay Health Foundation (among other groups) performs a similar function.

Suddenly, lesbian health initiatives are happening around the globe. In Canada the Michigan Organization for Human Rights funded a major health survey of 1681 lesbians, which gathered a wealth of useful information about lesbian health concerns. In 1992 the journal *Health Care for Women International* published a special issue on lesbian health which proved so popular that it was almost immediately reissued as a book, and there is now a small but steadily growing body of books on lesbian health in the publishers' catalogues. At least health care professionals can no longer make the excuse that information on lesbian health is not available!

Of course, this is just a beginning. It is still a fight to get funds for research into lesbian health, and there is a long way to go before lesbians are recognized as a client group with specific needs. There are still more questions than answers about lesbian health, and lesbians still meet with hostility and ignorance from health care workers on a regular basis. But there is cause for optimism.

Some important questions about lesbian health

During the months of research involved in writing this book, several key themes emerged time and time again. I'm adding them in here in the hope that somebody out there reading this will have the time, energy and resources to take them up!

First, we badly need answers to the question of whether or not lesbians are more vulnerable than non-lesbian women to breast cancer. Surprisingly, we do not in fact have any hard information on this one yet, despite alarmist reporting in the lesbian press and increasing concern among lesbian communities. All we know is that there are certain factors which appear to increase your risk of contracting breast cancer, and that some of these factors *we would expect* to be more common among lesbians. These factors are: not having had any children, having given birth relatively late in life, not having breastfed a child, high alcohol consumption and being overweight. Some experts have assumed that lesbians are more likely than non-lesbian women to be childless, but it would take very large-scale and complex research to prove this. What we do know is that giving birth in your twenties and breastfeeding your baby for as long as possible will offer some protection against breast cancer. This is *not* the same thing as saying that being a lesbian puts you at greater risk of developing breast cancer. There is also some evidence to suggest that, in some parts of the world (notably the USA), lesbians are more likely than non-lesbian women to be overweight, to abuse some street drugs and to drink excessive amounts of alcohol. These are, of course, risk factors for many other health problems as well as cancers; if lesbians are indeed more prone to these behaviours than are non-lesbian women, we need research which will tell us why and how these problems can be prevented.

This leads on to the second research issue, which is the larger question of the effects of homophobia on the self-esteem of lesbians. This is a complex question which may include issues as diverse as substance use or dependency, self-injury, eating disorders, obesity, suicide, battering in lesbian relationships, and depression or anxiety. Many of these questions are made more complex by the ways in which lesbian communities have responded to them. For example, we have seen that the question of obesity is a very difficult one for lesbians to address. Moreover, lesbian cultural and political values may have a complex influence on the way in which different lesbians perceive obesity. If it *is* true that a disproportionate number of lesbians are obese, what cultural factors specific to lesbians may account for this? Is it because lesbians are less bound up with pleasing a man, or because overeating is one response to the stress of confronting homophobia on a daily basis, or is it simply that lesbians appear to be fatter than non-lesbian women because of differences in clothing style or because public lesbian events are more welcoming of fat women than public heterosexual events? It quickly becomes clear, when thinking about such questions, that homophobia is not simply something which has an impact on individuals; rather, it must be understood as something which shapes our cultures, communities and belief systems.

Perhaps the most surprising area of neglect in lesbian health research is mental health. Feminists have pinpointed heterosexuality as one major cause of emotional and psychological distress in women,[16] so we might anticipate that being a lesbian offers a degree of protection against the commonest expressions of distress in women, such as anxiety and depression. On the other hand, living from day to day in a homophobic society must surely have an impact on the emotional and psychological wellbeing of lesbians? Unfortunately, the bulk of what is written about lesbian mental health concentrates on alcohol and substance misuse and on lesbian relationship issues. There is an extraordinary amount of attention paid to lesbian partner battering (an important issue, but for some reason one which receives a disproportionate amount of concern) and to pseudo-issues like 'merger' and 'lesbian bed death', which make special lesbian problems out of universally common human experiences. Yet there are many lesbians for whom 'mental health' means struggling to deal with the psychiatric system and with profoundly distressing experiences of depression, confusion, overwhelmingly powerful feelings or delusions or hallucinations. What relationship, if any, is there between these women's painful experiences and their lesbianism? Ironically, much lesbian energy which has gone into setting up alternatives to the psychiatric system for distressed women or into mental health activism has gone unrecognized. Little attention has been paid to the specific mental health needs of lesbians, or to the kinds of services which might best support lesbians who are severely disabled by psychological distress.

This wish-list of lesbian health research issues could easily go on for pages. Suffice it to say that writing a health handbook for lesbians will be much easier once we have some clear answers to at least some of these questions. It is likely that being a lesbian is, in general, good for your health. Several surveys have shown that lesbians are more psychologically 'well' than non-lesbian women, that we cope with relationship break-up better, that we have fewer sexually transmitted diseases and that we are more likely to report a high level of satisfaction with our sex lives. It is likely that homophobia can be identified as the major threat to lesbian health and wellbeing, responsible for our disproportionately high rates of alcoholism, suicide and obesity, and for the widespread use of therapy in some lesbian communities. In the chapters that follow, the consequences of homophobia emerge as an important element in every aspect of lesbian health. One thing we can say with certainty about lesbian health is that it is a political issue.

Further reading

Regan McClure and Anne Vespry (eds), *Lesbian Health Guide* (Toronto: Queer Press, 1994). Lesbian-specific health handbook, with a lesbian-feminist slant.

Cuca Hepburn and Bonnie Gutierrez, *Alive and Well: A Lesbian Health Guide* (Freedom, California: Crossing Press 1988). Ditto.

Phyllis Noerager Stern (ed.), *Lesbian Health: What are the Issues?* (London: Taylor and Francis, 1993). Collection of research articles on lesbian health.

Boston Women's Health Book Collective (eds), *The New Our Bodies Ourselves: A Health Book By and For Women*, British edition edited by Angela Phillips and Jill Rakusen (Harmondsworth: Penguin, 1989). Huge and extraordinarily detailed women's health handbook, with good lesbian section.

Evelyn C. White, *The Black Women's Health Book: Speaking for Ourselves* (Seattle: Seal Press, 1990). Black women's health handbook with some discussion of lesbian issues. Some of the chapters (including the only chapter on lesbian health) have been reprinted in Melba Wilson, *Healthy and Wise: The Essential Health Handbook for Black Women* (London: Virago, 1994), which has a British perspective.

Networking

Britain

LesBeWell: lesbian health group based in Birmingham which publishes a regular health newsletter for lesbians, *Dykenosis*, and a *Research Network Update* for lesbian health researchers. Contact them at: LesBeWell, PO Box 4048, Moseley, Birmingham B13 8DP.

Women's Health Information Centre (information on a vast range of women's health issues, including lesbian issues): 52–4 Featherstone Street, London EC1Y 8RT.

Royal College of Nursing Lesbian and Gay Working Party (for research into nursing issues and support of lesbian and gay nurses) can be contacted at: Royal College of Nursing, 20 Cavendish Square, London W1M 0AB.

USA

The National Lesbian and Gay Health Foundation Inc., PO Box 65472, Washington DC 20035.

Boston Women's Health Book Collective (for pamphlets, workshops and factsheets on different health issues): 240A M Street, Davis Square, Somerville, MA 02114.

National Women's Health Network (distributes an information pack on lesbian health issues and runs a comprehensive health information service): 514 10th Street, N.W., Ste 400, Washington DC 20004.

Europe

Women's Global Network for Reproductive Rights (useful newsletter and resource library): NZ Voorburgwal 32, 1012 RZ Amsterdam, The Netherlands.

2 The Basics: Maintaining Good Health

There are many reasons why lesbians might find it difficult to maintain good health. First, and most obviously, there are the daily stresses of living in a society which is openly hostile to lesbians. For many of us these stresses are compounded by a daily struggle against racism, poverty and a widespread failure to recognize and meet the needs of elderly lesbians or disabled women. Many of these issues have a very direct impact on our mental or emotional wellbeing, and are dealt with in later chapters. However, they also have indirect consequences for physical health.

For a start, lesbians are women. This means that we are disadvantaged in terms of employment and income. Many (though not all) heterosexual women are less acutely affected by this, since, if they are partnered by men and have access to a male wage, they will also enjoy all the benefits of heterosexual coupling, such as the protection of pension schemes, insurance benefits, etc. Two lesbians in a long-term relationship generally have to survive on a lower income, even if both partners are working, and will not have automatic protection from each other's work-related pension or insurance schemes. This means that lesbians are more likely to be living in poverty than heterosexual women of their own social class, age and ethnic group, and poverty has a very negative impact on health and on the kinds of health care available to you.

Second, the facilities for leisure and socializing which the heterosexual world takes for granted are simply not available on equal terms to lesbians. Pubs, bars, restaurants, cinemas, sports and leisure centres, cafés, theatres and concert venues are all places where heterosexuals can relax and unwind with their friends and partners. Most of them are places where it is simply not safe for a lesbian to be with her girlfriend. If you do sit with your arm around her, kiss her or hold her hand, it is often out of bravado or a refusal to be cowed, or a tentative experiment to see whether it will be OK this time, in this particular place. It is almost never the unselfconscious gesture of affection which heterosexual couples take completely for granted. This is exhausting, and is the main reason why we need our own spaces to relax in. Unfortunately, almost all the lesbian or lesbian and gay safe spaces are bars or clubs. They revolve around consuming alcohol and/or recreational drugs and are often smoke-filled and noisy. There is a well-established tradition in the United States and Canada of substance-free social spaces or events for lesbians, a tradition which has limited support in the (much smaller) lesbian communities in Britain and other European countries, but the substance-free ethos can be restricting. We seem all too often to be trapped between two extremes: the noisy, druggy, smoky disco on the one hand and the puritanically substance-free wimmin's music event on the other. It is hardly surprising that so much research suggests that lesbians have particular problems with alcohol and other substance use.

Finally, exercise is essential to maintaining good health. This is true for everyone, at whatever age and however able-bodied. Yet taking regular exercise can pose particular problems for lesbians. Membership of a private gym or sports club is expensive, and many local council or YMCA facilities do not recognize the needs of their lesbian clientele. Gyms can be daunting places, either crammed with smelly, sweaty men[1] or full of girly straight women in pink lycra and big hairdos trying to tone and firm for their boyfriends. In places where lesbian communities are large enough to support a softball or football or hockey team, those of us who are into team sports can have lots of good healthy fun, but this doesn't meet the needs of everyone.

The effects of living in a lesbian-hostile society influence our relationships to food, recreational drugs and exercise. Since these are the basic ingredients of good health, we need to think carefully about what steps we can take to protect our health in spite of social factors which we can do little about.

Your body or your life: can you be healthy and have fun?

All too often health education makes it seem as if we have to choose between health and pleasure. Good health, it appears, comes at the expense of consuming the food and drink we like, enjoying the leisure pursuits that appeal or taking solace from anything which goes by the suspect name of 'substance'. Yet this is the case only if you think of your body as a machine and 'health' in a very limited way. According to this idea of health the only healthy person is one who is her 'ideal' weight, devours appropriate quantities of the 'right' foods and none of the 'wrong' ones, indulges in wholesome and health-promoting leisure activities and gets her thrills from introducing a new herbal tea into her life or trying on some new fluorescent lycra number for increased performance at the gym (rather than greater success down at the disco). This idea is, in itself, damaging to the self-esteem and health potential of many lesbians, since the realities of homophobia mean that we are more likely to turn to 'forbidden pleasures' for solace. Health promotion advice which ignores this simply excludes lesbians.

In fact, health is infinitely more complex than this. The World Health Organization defines health as 'a state of complete physical, mental and social wellbeing and not merely the absence of disease or infirmity'.[2] Moreover, recent research into the workings of the immune system point to an immensely subtle and still enigmatic relationship between physical, emotional and social factors which appear to act together to protect us from ill health (or not). It is debatable, for example, whether a woman whose entire life is expended in the miserable business of obsessive dieting and exercising in order to achieve her so-called ideal weight may be accurately thought of as 'healthy'. Health is about creating the individual balance which enables each one of us to be comfortable and safe in the world, to resist disease and to live and enjoy our lives as fully as possible. No behaviour or activity is *intrinsically* 'healthy': most exercise carries the risk of injury, no food is health-giving on its own, and giving up an unhealthy habit such as smoking, binge-eating or drinking coffee may be very stressful.

Most writers on lesbian health agree that it is extremely difficult for lesbians to be comfortable and safe in a world that is so openly hostile to us. Stress, generally accepted to be a highly significant factor in an increasing number of illnesses, is likely to be experienced more often by people who experience prejudice and discrimination on a daily basis. Black women, for example, recognize that 'Stress-related illness . . . is a direct result of . . . the racist and sexist environment in which we live. For Black women . . . understanding and learning to deal with stress is a matter of personal survival and political necessity'.[3] For lesbians, confronting the daily reality of homophobia means inevitable stress, and this must be taken into account when thinking about how we may maintain our health.

The limits to personal responsibility: out of our control

It would be possible for lesbians to be one hundred per cent healthy only in a society which loved, respected and took good care of its lesbian members, which was free of racism, sexism and class inequality, which was fully accessible to and supportive of people with physical or intellectual impairments, and where environmental toxins and pollutants were unknown. Clearly many of the things which make good health possible are completely out of our control. Indeed, it is probably true to say that most of the factors which promote or damage health are social, cultural or political in nature. This is why it is so inadequate (and insulting) of health educators, governments and others to insist that we can all take responsibility for our health. Not true! However, given the right information and appropriate support, there are ways in which we as individuals can act to preserve or improve our health within the limits of our lives.

Please do not regard the information in this chapter as a set of instructions. It is not the case that if you take up all these suggestions you will become a healthy lesbian. However, what it will give you is the basic information you may find useful in determining what you want to do to take the best possible care of yourself.

Food

Worldwide the greatest problem associated with food is simply how to get enough of it to stay alive and well. In the developed nations the picture is more complex, with a (growing) minority of people too poor to feed themselves adequately, a larger minority too poor to feed themselves well, and conspicuous over-consumption by many of processed foods with little or no nutritional value. It is probably true to say that very few people eat 'well'. Many lesbians live in communities which support alternative health-promoting diets; the set of values which goes along with lesbian feminism, for example, tends to include an awareness of issues such as vegetarianism or the dangers of agrochemicals and food additives. However, many lesbians live in low-income households and simply cannot afford 'healthy' foods, which are often more expensive than the less healthy alternative. Still others may simply not have much information about healthy eating, while some younger urban dykes may have grown up regarding junk foods as the norm (or as fun to eat) and see no reason to change. So what exactly constitutes 'healthy' eating and why does it matter?

There is a mountain of evidence linking certain foods – animal and dairy fats, refined sugars and red meat – to life-threatening diseases such as cancers, heart disease or strokes. However, if you want to know *how much* of certain foods is likely to be harmful, or *how long* you have to eat them before they damage your health, the evidence is much less clear. Moreover, foods such as whole milk or butter do have nutritional value, and any drastic attempt to cut a specific food out of your diet may have unforeseen negative consequences. What we can say with confidence is that cutting down on your consumption of 'harmful' foods won't do any harm and is very likely to protect your health.

When it comes to food additives, there is increasingly worrying evidence linking a whole range of them to an equally wide range of disorders, from allergies and mood disorders to cancers and birth defects. There are thousands of food additives, and becoming obsessive about them is probably not very good for your mental health – a good rule of thumb is simply to avoid them as far as you can, given the kind of life you lead. If you pop out for a burger and chips every lunch time, try a take-away from a local health food store two or three times a week instead, or make yourself a sandwich with wholemeal bread.

Put at its simplest, these guidelines will help you eat well

Take plenty of:

- *fresh fruit and vegetables*. These are rich in vitamins and minerals and there is evidence that they protect against cancers and reduce the risk of heart disease. You should aim for five or more portions a day, cook them as little as possible, and eat as wide a variety as possible. Dark green leafy vegetables also contain calcium, which is useful if you cannot tolerate milk. Moreover, many fruits and vegetables provide fibre, which is essential to the health of the gut.

- *complex carbohydrates*. These can be found in grain products such as pasta, rice or wholemeal bread. They give energy in a form which the body can use readily, and are filling without being fattening. Athletes eat a lot of complex carbohydrates. Again, wholemeal bread and oat bran are good sources of fibre, though there is evidence that wheat bran can move too quickly through the gut.

- *protein-rich foods*. Protein is essential to good health. It is found in seeds (sesame seeds, sunflower seeds, etc.), pulses (lentils and beans), milk, cheese and eggs, meat, fish, brown rice, tofu, quorn products, nuts and wholemeal bread. There is evidence that oily fish (such as mackerel or sardines) are particularly good for you and, as they are a source of protein as well, it is a good idea to include them in your regular diet.

- *water*. Water is essential to life, and drinking plenty can improve digestion, flush toxins and waste from the system, and result in clearer skin and better general health. If you drink your water in the form of tea or coffee, don't forget that you are taking in toxins along with the water. Coffee has been linked to non-malignant breast disease, miscarriage, high blood pressure, osteoporosis, pre-menstrual problems and problems with kidneys and bladder (although some recent evidence suggests that drinking one or two cups a day is unlikely to cause significant health problems).[4] Steer clear of canned soft drinks, which contain sugars, additives and caffeine. You don't have to drink bottled mineral water either (there is some evidence to suggest that drinking too much can lead to kidney and bladder problems), though you may like to buy a simple jug filter to filter impurities such as heavy metals and other toxins out of your tap water.

Go easy on:

- *fats*. The evidence about whether butter or margarine is better for you is complex and contradictory, so you are probably best advised to use what you prefer for spreading. Just use it in moderation. For cooking, use vegetable oils rather than lard or dripping. Olive oil is expensive, but it seems to offer some protection against heart disease so it is worthwhile economizing on other things in order to use it if at all possible. If you can afford it, other oils such as sesame seed oil or walnut oil can add exciting flavour to stir-fries and other cooking, and will add variety to your intake of vitamins.

- *processed foods*. There is little point trying to avoid processed foods altogether, unless you are the kind of person who finds it easy to put a lot of time and energy into monitoring what you eat. However, it is worth trying to eat them as little as possible within the demands of your lifestyle. They often contain little of nutritional value, and most will give you a good dose of chemical additives with under-researched side effects on your long-term health.

- *salt*. While salt is essential to good health, we require only a trace of it, and most of us eat far too much. It is added to most processed foods in quite extravagant quantity. Too much salt can lead to high blood pressure, water retention and other problems. Don't cook with salt, try to add less to your meals and become conscious of how much is 'hidden' in snacks and convenience foods.

There is only one 'food' which you should avoid altogether, and that is sugar. Of course it is almost impossible to avoid sugar since manufacturers put it into everything from baked beans to toothpaste, and most of us find life a lot easier and more fun with the occasional indulgence in a sticky bun, slab of chocolate or mug of sweet coffee. Just remember that sugar has no nutritional value at all and that it really is not good for you. It is up to you to weigh this up with the psychological benefits to be gained from your personal sugar 'hit'.

In general, nutritionists recommend that you eat between five and twelve servings of grain products a day (bread, bagels, pasta, rice and cereals), between five and ten servings of fresh vegetables and fruit, two to four servings of dairy produce (milk, yoghurt, butter, cheese) and two or three servings of a protein-rich food (meat, poultry, fish, nuts, pulses). Using organic produce (meat and vegetables produced by traditional methods, without the use of chemicals) will ensure that you keep your intake of harmful substances to a minimum. Organic produce is now widely available in many supermarkets as well as in specialist shops, and it really does taste better!

You may be tempted to take a short cut to good nutrition in the form of vitamin tablets or other supplements. Be warned that this approach has problems. There is evidence that getting vitamins and minerals in fresh food is better for you than taking them in tablet form. Our bodies have evolved to make the best use of natural foods, and the specific combinations of vitamins, minerals and other substances in those foods seem to be important. It is also possible to overdose on some vitamins and minerals. What is more, taking vitamin pills will not compensate for the harm that can be done by processed foods in other ways (such as the toxic effects of chemical additives).

Cost

One major problem with 'healthy' foods is that they tend to be more expensive than the mass-produced alternatives. Wholemeal bread, for example, usually costs more than ready-sliced, plastic-wrapped additive-rich white bread. If you are on a tight budget you can make your money go further by a few simple tricks:

- Shop at local markets, farm shops and greengrocers for your fruit and veg. They may not have the same range as the big supermarkets, but prices are often lower.

- Do your supermarket shopping late on Saturday or Sunday, when there are often big reductions in fresh food which needs to be sold before the new week's stock is put on the shelves. There are almost always special reductions on foods close to their sell-by date.

- Try growing some vegetables or fruit in your garden, or even in a window-box. I once grew a healthy crop of tomatoes on my bedsit window-sill, but runner beans, spinach, radishes or little lettuces will do just as well as tomatoes in a large pot or window-box, and all can be grown cheaply from seed. Even the smallest garden has room for an apple tree. They grow well in tubs, although planting them in the ground works better. You can buy young trees which have two or three different species of apple grafted on to them, and these can be very fruitful. A herb garden can be established on any window-sill for very little money, and herbs are a good source of trace minerals.

- Ask friends who grow vegetables if you can have surplus produce, or offer to buy some cheaply. In Britain, rent an allotment from the local council, or consider co-renting one with a friend if you don't have the time to spare to maintain one yourself.

- Get into sprouting alfalfa and/or chick peas. This is simply done in old glass jars with a little water. You don't need fancy bean-sprouting equipment, although you can buy special plastic containers if you have the money to spare. The resultant sprouts are delicious and highly nutritious, go well in salads and sandwiches or in stir-fries, and are really cheap.

- Experiment with cheap foods which may be new to you, such as lentils, different types of beans or different breads. Specialist ethnic food shops in large cities often sell traditional foods much more cheaply than local supermarkets, and are usually willing to advise on preparation and cooking. Whatever your own cultural background, other cultures have much to offer in the way of foods which have been nourishing people for centuries! Try Chinese, Indian, Pakistani or Jewish supermarkets, and Caribbean or Bangladeshi corner shops.

Making changes in your eating

Food is important to our emotional security and familiar ways of eating, however 'unhealthy' they may look to a health educator, may be useful in maintaining emotional health. Aim for small, gradual changes in what you eat. This will allow your body time to adjust and you time to become familiar with new tastes and cooking habits. This caution is difficult, however, if you have just decided to become a vegetarian (eating a meat-free diet) or a vegan (eating no animal produce at all, including milk, cheese or eggs). Once you have decided that, for ethical or other reasons, you are going to stop eating certain foods altogether, you cannot take that step gradually. Vegetarian cooking is becoming more popular generally, especially among some lesbian feminist communities, so there should be little difficulty in getting good advice about how to replace the protein, vitamins and minerals you have been getting from meat. Being vegan is more difficult, since it involves quite detailed knowledge about how foods work in combination to provide all the nourishment essential to life and health. *If you intend to become vegan, you must learn how to do it well*. Buy a book, get in touch with other vegans who can give you advice, and be prepared for the fact that you may experience some quite dramatic effects from this dramatic change in your eating. You may lose a lot of weight, pre-menopausal women may find their periods stop for a while, and you may get diarrhoea, constipation or wind.

Eating and body-image

The issue of eating is never simple. Food carries with it in every culture a complicated package of social, emotional and cultural meanings. For women in the industrial nations of the West there are huge emotional issues associated with the purchase, preparation and eating of food, as well as with the expectation that women should feed everyone else. This means that the most obvious food-related health issue, weight, is far from simple.

The belief that health equals slimness has powerful support from the medical industry. Certainly it is the case that being overweight is potentially very harmful – if you want to find out just how harmful, tuck in to any diet book. Weight is also a potent political issue. Feminists rightly point to a manipulative diet industry, which exploits women's fears about their physical health and their sexual attractiveness for profit, and to the political implications of a cultural 'norm', which insists that women should sacrifice time, energy, money and often their health in the interests of slenderness.

Despite these concerns, it remains the case that being more than a little overweight is potentially damaging to anyone's health and wellbeing, while being seriously overweight may be extremely harmful and certainly shortens life. However, what counts as 'overweight' is not necessarily easy to define, and the physical risks of being fat may need to be balanced against the hazards of many dieting behaviours and any psychological *benefits* which the fat woman gains from her fat. The woman who carries around a potentially health-damaging load of excess body-fat may need to be big in order to protect her emotional health – being fat and taking up space may be the easiest way for a woman to feel powerful or protected in a hostile world which denigrates and 'belittles' women, or the fat may be acting as a necessary security blanket or suit of armour, protecting an unbearable sense of vulnerability.

However, the health risks associated with being fat are not solely physical. The psychological costs may be very damaging. Autobiographical accounts of fat lesbians make it clear that the stresses associated with the social and cultural condemnation of fat people – never finding clothes you like in your size, being perceived as ugly or asexual, experiencing contempt and disgust from other people – can be extremely painful. As one woman grimly explains, 'My "safe space" is in my bed with a book. Beyond that, it's pretty risky.'[5]

The relationship of body mass to self-esteem, emotional safety and physical health is so complex that it is simply not possible to generalize. This section does not assume that all lesbians want to lose weight. Indeed, there are perfectly valid reasons for wanting to *increase* weight: elderly people who are very thin are less able to survive illness and surgery, and there is growing evidence that being *underweight* carries its own health risks. What it does assume is that most lesbians wish to 'manage' their weight – that is, not to control it but to work towards a state of equilibrium where your body mass, whether large or small, supports rather than damages your physical and emotional health. This balance is a complex one, and you are the only person who can decide what body size best contributes to your physical and emotional equilibrium.

By and large, weight is fairly directly associated with food intake. There are, of course, some medical conditions which make it impossible for some women to be anything other than fat, whatever they eat. However, such conditions are relatively rare and, if you have reason to believe that you have such a condition, you may be able to work with your health advisers to reduce their effect on your body mass. Such clinically identifiable malfunctions are quite distinct from simply having an inherited tendency to put on weight easily which, although making it harder to manage your weight, may be balanced by relatively small changes in your eating.

If you are unhappy with your body-image

There may be lesbians who are joyfully celebratory about every inch of their bodies, but such a happy state almost certainly requires long-term hard work on an emotional level. Research repeatedly indicates that most women would like to be thinner and, although many lesbian communities are more accepting of a wider range of body shapes and sizes than the heterosexual mainstream, there is no doubt that many lesbians are unhappy with their body-image and especially that many of us think we are too fat.[6] If you want to be thinner you have three options. You can work at learning to accept your body at the size and shape it is, you can adopt a formal diet plan and work to achieve a 'target' weight, or you can change your eating habits in a way that suits you and that you are confident that you can maintain and see what happens to your weight.

Whichever you choose, first make sure that you really are overweight. This is not as easy as it sounds. I once lost five stone in weight, but my reflection in the mirror didn't look any smaller to me, and the only way I could believe in what the scales told me was to keep putting my new size 12 self back into my old size 20 jeans. Much has been written about the experience of women with eating disorders, who may perceive themselves as fat when they are life-threateningly thin, but researchers are increasingly coming to recognize that very few people can look in a mirror and make an accurate assessment of their body size. Before you make any attempt to lose weight it may be a good idea to check out with a few trusted friends, your doctor or complementary practitioner whether you are in fact 'overweight'. If you feel very uneasy at doing this, or if you know that you simply will not believe anyone who says you are not overweight, consider the possibility that something may be going on for you at an emotional level which you need to look at before launching on any changes to your eating. It is useful for all of us to recognize that concentrating on the way we look may be a way of dealing with painful issues which are less easy to control. It is not difficult to understand how we may react to the pain of living in a world that hates and despises us by attempting to control our appearance. Some lesbians may decide that they can express their freedom from the need to be sexually attractive to men by allowing themselves to put on as much weight as they want. Or they may decide that they want to show the world that not all lesbians are the 'fat, ugly man-haters' of the offensive stereotype by being as slim and conventionally attractive as they can. Or they may simply respond to a culture which makes lesbians invisible by taking up as much physical space as possible.

Such survival strategies in the teeth of homophobia come on top of all the issues which confront non-lesbian as well as lesbian women. Issues such as a history of sexual or physical abuse, experience of sexual violence or abusive partnerships may all find expression in attempts to control body size:

Body image problems can be seen as coping strategies to deal with stresses, strong emotions and painful experiences . . . Often a woman's body becomes a vehicle to play out issues of control and powerlessness. Controlling her body may become a substitute for not having control in other areas of her life.[7]

Only you can decide, weighing up the reasons why you want to be lighter and balancing them against the reasons why you may have become heavier than you want to be, that you need to lose some weight. Once you have made that decision, you will do it. If you have any remaining uncertainties, it is unlikely that you will succeed in losing weight, and you may find yourself on the depressing treadmill of loss/gain which so many dieters get stuck on.

How to lose weight

The watchwords, as with any change in lifestyle, are *gently does it*. Suddenly and dramatically reducing your food intake will make you feel ill, exhausted and dizzy, and will do you no good at all. Similarly, cutting favourite foods out of your diet may be depressing and difficult to maintain. If you follow the healthy eating guidelines above, you will at least know that your body is getting what it needs to function properly.

The key to losing weight is simple. Eat less! In particular, eat fewer foods which contain fat and/or sugar. You may find that simply reducing the portions you eat will be enough. Where you would normally have four roast potatoes with a meal, have two. Where you would normally have a large helping of chocolate chip ice cream, have a much smaller helping. Aim to cut sweets, salty snacks and chocolate out of your diet as much as possible *eventually*. But recognize the emotional needs which are being met by treats such as chocolate, and work out how you can reduce your consumption of these sources of comfort rather than abandon them altogether. For example, if you recognize that you binge on chocolate a few days before your period starts, you can restrict your chocolate intake to those few days. By *accepting* that chocolate is useful to you during that time, you can balance out your use of chocolate as an emotional resource. The same emotional factors can help you decide whether to make use of diet aids or to join slimming clubs. Diet aids and slimming clubs are expensive and not necessary to losing weight. However, if you are the kind of person who responds well to imposed discipline or to ritual, you may feel that they would be appropriate for you.

Please remember that going on a diet is *not* a good way to manage your weight. Once you come off the diet, you will be back at square one, and the constant increase and decrease of weight involved can be harmful to your health. What you are aiming for is a *permament change in your eating pattern*. You have to decide that you are going to eat like this for the rest of your life, so there is no point trying to live on lettuce and cottage cheese. Be flexible, reducing some foods bit by bit, increasing your use of others, cutting out only those foods you can really live without, and allowing yourself to use food as comfort or celebration from time to time. If you have been used to eating four potatoes with your evening meal, a slice of chocolate gateau with your lunch and three sweet biscuits with your morning coffee, you could replace lunch with a diet drink, supper with a lettuce leaf and half a radish, and drink your morning coffee black with no sugar and no edible treat at all. And that would be hell. Much better to stick to your preferred foods and just *cut down*; two potatoes rather than four, a much thinner slice of gateau (or a piece of fruit) and just one sweet biscuit. That, you can live with!

How to gain weight

If you want to gain weight, you can do this safely by gradually increasing your consumption of starchy foods like pasta, tortillas and potatoes. Do not feel that you have to reach for the sugary or fatty foods that are the despair of your dieting sisters, since these foods are not healthy. You may also wish to increase the amount of protein-rich foods that you eat, and to change your drinking habits. If you are trying to gain weight, try drinking a pint of beer with a meal rather than two glasses of wine, or a milkshake (made with fresh fruit and real ice cream of course!) rather than a cup of coffee.

Exercise: does it have to hurt?

Whether you are trying to lose weight or to gain it, the right kind of exercise can help. Aerobic exercise helps burn off fat, while muscle-building exercise can increase your muscle-to-fat ratio, which (because muscle is denser than fatty tissue) will increase your weight as well as making you stronger. And don't forget that weight-bearing exercises will help build up your bone density, which offers some protection against osteoporosis in later life, something which is likely to be especially important to underweight women.

If you have the idea that getting healthy exercise involves complex time- and money-consuming activities requiring expensive clothing and specialist equipment, think again! Although it can be very rewarding on many levels to take your exercise this seriously, many lesbians simply do not have the time or money to do so, or may simply not be interested. Yet regular exercise is very good for you. However old you are, and whatever your physical abilities, exercise is important for general health, keeping your body strong and supple, and you feeling happy. Recent research has shown that even very elderly people can improve their general fitness and mobility with regular exercise, and it is so beneficial in terms of stress relief and mood improvement that psychologists and psychiatrists have begun to prescribe exercise to people suffering from clinical depression. Exercise can burn off the adrenaline which our bodies produce in response to stress, so can be very helpful in anxiety, insomnia and many stress-related illnesses.

If you have not exercised for a long time, start gently and seek the advice of your doctor or alternative practitioner about what kinds of exercise would be best for you. You also need to think about what you spend most of your time doing. If you stand on your feet all day, for example, swimming or yoga will be more appealing and probably of more benefit to you than activities such as running or dancing. If you are cooped up in an office all day, it may be more fun and more useful to go for a swim or a walk during your lunch break than to try and find the energy and motivation to go out in the evening after the day's work.

There are four main physical benefits of exercise

- *Stimulation of heart and lungs*. Activities that do this are called *aerobic* exercises, and require vigorous and sustained activity of your large muscles. To improve the function of your heart and lungs you must regularly do exercise that is strenuous enough to increase your heart rate and get you out of breath. If you have a heart condition or breathing difficulties (such as asthma or chronic bronchitis), you should begin such activities under reliable supervision. 'Aerobics' classes offer supervised exercise designed to improve heart and lung function and general fitness, but they can be daunting. Fast walking, gentle running, swimming, skipping, kick-boxing or dancing are all good. Dancing can mean disco dancing, but can just as well be ballroom, country line dancing, folk dancing or prancing around in private to the strains of your personal stereo. If you have young children, you can get quite a bit of aerobic exercise by playing vigorous games with them. If you are an older lesbian or if you have mobility impairment, seek advice on aerobic activities which are within your capabilities.

- *Flexibility*. Keeping muscles supple and joints flexible is important at any age and at any level of physical ability. Stretching exercises, such as yoga or tai chi, help you recover from or prevent injury, and can also improve blood supply to internal organs. You should *always* warm up with stretching exercises before taking part in heavy physical activities such as weight training, running or team games. Any sports instructor should be able to give you a full programme of stretching exercises, or you can find them in most exercise instruction manuals.

- *Strength*. You can increase the strength of both your muscles and your bones. For women, maintaining bone mass is important, as it helps prevent osteoporosis. This is a condition which affects many women after the menopause (because of the reduction in the amount of oestrogen circulating in the blood) and results in brittle bones, which are vulnerable to fractures and joint injury. Exercises which increase strength in bones and muscles include working out with weights, rock climbing, gymnastics and most water sports (because of having to work against the drag effect of the water). If you are starting weight training or gymnastics, do so with a properly qualified instructor and start off gently.

- *Balance and co-ordination*. Activities which involve hitting, kicking or catching a ball will all improve co-ordination, while anything that gets you to move in a pre-determined way (dancing, tai chi, yoga, etc.) will improve co-ordination and balance.

Any increase in physical activity will also result in an increase in your overall level of energy and in your resistance to infection (especially important for people with mobility impairments), an improvement in your mood, better sleep, relaxation and an increase in stamina. You will feel less stressed, less fatigued and more resiliant. Go to it!

As with every piece of advice in this chapter, the important word is *gently*! You do *not* have to 'feel the burn' in order to get benefit from exercise. Nor does it have to hurt to prove it is doing you good. Indeed, apart from the pleasant ache of well-used muscles, pain is a sign that there is something wrong or that your are overdoing it. Start simply, and you will be surprised how quickly you feel able to do that bit more and go that bit further. It is also important to choose the kind of exercise which you can enjoy. Don't join the local women's football team if you hated team games at school and are filled with cynicism about the idea of 'team spirit'. Similarly, don't expect to be happy working out down at the gym on your own if you are a bubbly, sociable type. Do not exercise if you are not eating properly (your body needs to be able to burn available food resources), and make sure you drink plenty to allow for sweating. Don't drink alcohol in conjunction with exercise (it can dehydrate you) and don't gulp down a pint of juice ten minutes before you begin – either drink a substantial amount about half an hour before your exercise starts or take along a small bottle of water or juice and take *small sips* as your exercise. Don't use carbonated fizzy drinks (despite the advertising), as they can give you an unpleasant 'gassed-up' feeling.

The body beautiful? A note on exercise and body-image

It is hard to separate exercise from body-image. Many straight women exercise *only* in order to stay 'toned' and slim for their male partners (or to attract a male partner), and among some lesbian communities there is a decided bias in favour of an 'ideal' body shape which is firm, muscular and quite athletic-looking. Lesbians are probably able to go further than non-lesbian women in terms of developing strength and musculature without fearing that we are becoming less feminine or too butch. In addition, many (though not all) lesbian communities are less concerned to promote slimness than the mainstream culture, and are more happy to accept fat lesbians for what they are. Nevertheless, although these factors seem to give us more leeway than our heterosexual sisters, we should be aware that there *are* ideas circulating in our communities about what makes an attractive woman, and that these ideas are bound to have an impact on us. If you become aware that you are exercising (or, indeed, that you are *not* exercising) in order to conform to some ideal of lesbian beauty, remember that, although it is wonderful to have other women enjoying your body, *you* have the right to enjoy your own body in ways that suit you.

Substances: use and abuse

That word 'substance', as in 'substance-free' or 'substance abuse', carries some pretty loaded meanings for many lesbians and, increasingly, for lesbian communities. Some of those meanings have become quite punitive: it is seen as a Bad Thing for lesbians to abuse substances, and substance-free spaces are regarded by those who promote them as not only a Good Thing, but politically sound and necessary to the health of the Lesbian Nation. As, indeed, they are. However, a sizeable dollop of moralism has crept into the substances debate in some lesbian communities. One lesbian feminist has even gone on record as saying that coffee consumption is of the same order as sadomasochistic sexual practices (she finds both equally distasteful).[8] Because of this moralism, I prefer to use Lesley Doyal's term, 'drugs of solace'.[9]

The drugs of solace are those things which have little or no nutritional benefit yet which we turn to to make us feel good in an often depressing, dangerous, frustrating, enraging or simply mundane life. They all have the potential to damage our health to a greater or lesser degree, yet living without them is difficult in societies where their use is widely accepted, where much social interaction revolves around their use – the rituals surrounding the consumption of alcohol, coffee, nicotine or street drugs are an important part of their appeal – and where emotional survival can sometimes feel precarious. Moreover, if their effects were not enjoyable, nobody would use them anyway! So this is not going to be a 'just say no' lecture. Looking in turn at alcohol, tobacco, street drugs and coffee, it is possible to assess the more important health consequences of each, with no assumption that total abstinence is your personal goal. I have not addressed prescription drugs such as tranquillizers here. Prescription drugs are less easily available than other drugs of solace, doctors are more aware of the dangers of addiction than they used to be, and using a prescribed drug to treat depression or other emotional problems means viewing your problems as in some way medical. These are all issues which deserve more space than is available here.

Alcohol

Lesbians are regularly reported to have disproportionately high rates of alcoholism,[10] and many lesbians in North America are involved in the 'twelve-step' culture of recovery. In Europe, where twelve-step programmes are less influential and where lesbian communities are smaller, or in more remote rural areas in the USA or Canada, lesbians who experience problems with their use of alcohol are likely to be more isolated.

Alcohol is deeply embedded in the social fabric of Euro-American cultures, and it is not easy to be a non-drinker. Moreover, there is persuasive evidence that alcohol taken in moderation is beneficial to health. A glass of red wine with the evening meal is thought to be actively good for your health, though alcohol is a poison and can cause quite severe health problems if you drink too much of it. Women have a lower tolerance of alcohol than do men, since our bodies metabolize it faster and absorb it more readily. The recommended safe intake for women is therefore less than for men. Current guidelines suggest that women should drink no more than twenty-one units spread throughout a week, with a couple of completely alcohol-free days to allow the body to deal with alcohol-related toxins. A 'unit' is roughly the amount of alcohol contained in one glass of wine, a single measure of spirits, a small glass of fortified wine such as sherry or port, or a half pint of beer. However, strong beers, lagers or cider may contain up to two units in each half pint, and most cocktails contain three or four.

Heavy drinking, generally defined as thirty-five or more units a week on a regular basis, can quite quickly lead to serious damage to health. Conditions which are linked to this kind of drinking include cancers of the liver, breast, colon and rectum, and of the mouth and throat (especially in smokers), high blood pressure, heart failure, liver damage and kidney problems. Excess alcohol also damages the function of the immune system, which has implications for people with HIV and other immune system dysfunction, and can lead to obesity or infertility. For lesbians who are trying to conceive (see Chapter 4), avoiding alcohol may improve your chances of successful pregnancy. It is also important not to combine drinking with other drugs, whether prescribed or illegal, since many drugs, such as antibiotics or cold cures, may react badly with alcohol.

The occasional drunken binge in response to a special occasion – getting a new job or being dumped by your girlfriend both fall into this category – is unlikely to cause any long-term damage to your health, provided you get drunk in safe circumstances where you are not going to be driving, operating machinery or taking responsibility for young children. However, if you find you are getting drunk on a regular basis, or if you find it difficult to stay within the recommended twenty-one units a week for whatever reason, you should take a serious look at your use of alcohol. It is important not even to *begin* to fall into the trap of hiding or denying that you may have a problem, since this is one sure sign that you do! If you are even faintly concerned about your drinking, *talk to someone* about it. That someone can be a friend (though not someone that you regularly drink with, or who consumes a lot of alcohol themselves), doctor, counsellor or work colleague whose judgement you trust. It is up to you to judge when to talk to people you are emotionally involved with – lovers or family members – since any emotional relationship is bound to be affected by your drinking and you may need the support of people who are more detached if you are to assess the situation clearly and work out what, if anything, you should do.

If you do decide that you need to change the way you use alcohol it doesn't mean that you have to sign up for Al-Anon on the spot. First try making some changes in your life which will enable you to replace alcohol and move on. You could find alternative places to bars and pubs to meet and socialize, or you could try sticking to soft drinks six nights out of seven. If you drink at home, try other treats to unwind. Spend the money you save by not buying drink on tempting food, visits to the cinema or theatre, or on a ticket to visit a friend you haven't seen in a while. There are books to help you develop a better relationship with alcohol, and all of them contain useful suggestions for cutting down your consumption. However, it is probably a good idea to give yourself a time limit for this kind of self-motivated change. Tell yourself that, if you are still worried at the end of two months, you will get some help. Tell a trusted friend too, and make sure they know when the two months will be up, so that you can get their support if needed for the next stage.

If you do decide you need to get help, get in touch with your doctor or other health adviser, or ring one of the many alcohol advice and support groups. You may not be able to find a group designed for lesbians, or one which openly welcomes lesbian members, or even one which recognizes that lesbians exist. This doesn't have to be a problem – we are all used to dealing with the heterosexual majority – but it certainly *can* be. If it is, try getting in touch with a women's mental health self-help group in your area and asking their advice. They may be able to put you in touch with a known lesbian or lesbian-friendly group, or suggest resources to support you in establishing a group for lesbians locally.

Alcoholism still carries a great deal of stigma. It is associated with being inadequate or out of control, with not coping and with violent or just plain embarrassing behaviour. The stigma against women with alcohol problems is greater than against men. After all, getting drunk is one of the socially acceptable rites of passage for adult males in our society. You may also find that people are only too willing to decide that you have a drink problem because you are a lesbian (rather than because *they* and others like them are homophobic, for

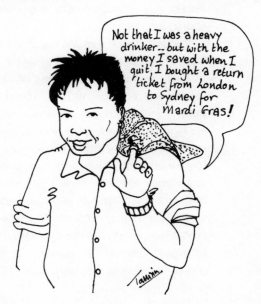

example!). Because of all this, admitting that you have a problem can be very difficult, and can bring with it feelings of failure and shame. But you have done nothing wrong. There is much evidence that a tendency to alcohol dependency is genetic for many people. Native Americans, for example, have a gene which makes it very difficult for their bodies to cope with alcohol. Even without a genetic predisposition, it is unsurprising that lesbians become addicted to alcohol in a society in which everybody (let alone lesbians) finds it difficult to live and which actively promotes the consumption of alcoholic drinks. The brewers spend unimaginable amounts of money to get you to buy their products, and you are not a bad person because you respond to all these pressures by drinking. On the other hand, don't use any of the above as an excuse to keep up a drink habit that you *know* is bad news.

Smoking

This one is tough! Whereas drinking in moderation can be good for you, *any* level of smoking is bad for you. But smokers know all that. You don't need me to tell you yet again about the lung cancer, the emphysema, the amputated limbs or jawbones, the mouth, tongue and throat cancers, the heart disease, the bladder and uterine cancers, the infertility, the low birth-weight babies and deaths from SIDS,[11] etc., etc. If you are a smoker, you *know* you should quit, and you probably want to. But not just yet.

There is absolutely no point at all in trying to quit smoking unless you want to. If you have doubts, it will be doubly difficult to cope with withdrawal. However, when you do want to give up, it needn't be the trauma you are expecting. There are dozens of books, videos and self-help groups which can support you in giving up, not to mention nicotine chewing gum, skin patches, hypnosis, acupuncture, etc., etc. The methods for quitting almost outnumber the diseases smoking gives you. So how is it different for lesbians?

First, because there is no doubt that smoking is a coping strategy in response to stress (albeit an unhelpful one), and lesbians have to deal with a lot of stress. Second, because not many support strategies recognize that lesbians exist. Third, because having a fag hanging out of your mouth is a useful stage prop if you are trying to establish butch cred, and a femme may feel ever so much more slinky with a slender cigarette between her fingers (forgetting, for a moment, that smokers smell and taste nauseating, that smoking makes your skin all thin and wrinkly, and that sucking on a fag is about as butch as sucking your thumb). And, finally, because we socialize in environments which are often smoky and positively reeking of the drug which you so desperately crave during withdrawal. However, there is also the fact that many lesbian feminist communities provide smoke-free events and spaces. If you do decide to quit, you may have to experiment with various support strategies or methods until you find one which works for you. But perhaps the most important thing to remember is that the beneficial effects of stopping smoking begin the minute you stub out your last ever cigarette. You will quite quickly find that your sense of smell and taste become sharper, and the damage that cigarettes have been doing to your health will begin to repair itself immediately. Of course, some of that damage may be irreparable, depending on how long you have been smoking and what harm has been done. However, research suggests that quitting can quickly start to reduce your risk of major smoking-associated illnesses, and the longer you stay off fags, the closer your health status will become to that of someone who has never smoked. If you smoke, giving up is the one thing you can do which will make the greatest improvement in your health and life chances.

Street drugs

Illegal drugs, or street drugs, tend to be associated with very specific subcultures. The dance culture around Ecstasy, for example, is very different from the street culture associated with heroin. Such subcultures tend to change over time as well. Marijuana use among the white counter-culture in the 1960s was of a very different order to its use among the African-Caribbean Rastafari, and different again to its current use among the educated middle classes in Europe and North America. There is no single street drug which is distinctively associated with lesbian culture in the way that alkyl nitrite ('poppers') is associated with gay men's disco culture. Yet lesbians may not be members of, or may lack access to, lesbian 'communities', or they may have loose ties to lesbian communities and closer ties to other communities structured around class, ethnicity or lifestyle. So we can be pretty certain that for every street drug there are lesbian users.

One major health concern relating to drug use is the method of delivery, that is whether you inject, smoke, snort or swallow the drug. Of the four, swallowing is not in itself a health risk but all the others are. Injecting is the most risky, not only because of the potential risk of acquiring HIV infection through sharing injecting equipment without cleaning but also because injecting carries the risk of infection, abscesses and ulceration and a nasty collection of blood-borne diseases such as hepatitis. To minimize such risks it is important either to have a supply of sterile needles and syringes for one use only (in Britain many drugs agencies and pharmacists run needle exchange projects) or to clean *all* injecting equipment thoroughly before and after each use. You don't have to use bleach (possession of bleach has been used by the police as evidence in court against drug users), since a thorough wash in a strong solution of ordinary dishwashing liquid in hot water (where possible) will be effective against most bacteria and against HIV. But equipment must be rinsed thoroughly with *clean* water afterwards, and needles and syringes flushed through three times with clean water, to avoid the risk of injecting washing-up liquid into your bloodstream. *Don't* share lubricating or rinsing water, cottons or cookers, and don't backload syringes.

Smoking a drug risks damage to the lungs, just as smoking tobacco does. Drugs that may be taken in other ways should not therefore be smoked, although smoking poses less short-term health risk than injecting. Chasing the dragon (smoking heroin) is less risky than injecting it, and eating cannabis resin (in cakes, cookies or Alice B. Toklas's famous fudge) is a less harmful alternative to smoking it. It is, however, less easy to regulate your intake if you eat a drug. If you are smoking it the effects are generally swift and you can stop smoking or take fewer drags as it starts to hit. Once you have eaten a fixed amount, it stays eaten, and you may find you have to deal with having taken more than you meant to. Sniffing or snorting can damage the nasal septum (the membrane between the nostrils) and the back of the throat. Also, sniffing volatile substances such as solvents makes it hard to control the amount you take.

There is not space here to detail the potential risks and effects of all street drugs. Such information is widely available elsewhere, and there is much information – both useful and misguided – circulating within drug-using peer groups. However, one health risk associated with all street drugs is their illegality. It is extremely stressful to be arrested, fined or imprisoned for possession of illegal drugs, and prison is *not* a health-promoting environment.

The Java jive:
how dangerous is coffee?

There has been much debate recently, in lesbian communities and in the mainstream media, concerning the health risks associated with coffee drinking. There is a long-standing tradition in some lesbian feminist circles of avoiding caffeine by drinking herbal teas, eating carob-bean products rather than chocolate and replacing coffee with a variety of grain-based beverages. It would not be ethically defensible for me to recommend these practices as healthier than drinking tea or coffee or eating chocolate, since there is no evidence to suggest that they are any better for you. However, coffee is an important part of many lesbians' lives, and there is a staggering body of research into the long-term effects of drinking coffee.[12]

Researchers agree that coffee is a stimulant, and that it is addictive. Users can become habituated, needing larger doses to get the desired effect, and giving up coffee may result in withdrawal symptoms which may include headaches and depression. Over-use – and individuals vary greatly in their sensitivity to all drugs, so one person's over-use may be fine for the next person – can lead to anxiety or agitation, insomnia, nausea and headaches. But what of the long-term hazards? Greatest concern has been expressed over the possibility that coffee drinking can increase the risk of heart disease, but millions of hours of research time have failed to come up with any conclusive evidence. What seems to be the case is that the amount your drink and the method you use to make your coffee may reduce any risk which does exist. Coffee prepared by the filter method contains very few of the substances suspected of increasing your risk of heart disease (lipids, associated with the production of cholesterol), whereas coffee made by any method that involves boiling (e.g. percolating it) contains far more of these substances. No coffee connoisseuse is going to boil her coffee anyway – 'coffee boiled is coffee spoiled' – and methods which leave the coffee to steep for a long time, such as the hot-plate used to keep coffee hot in some machines, also spoil the taste, so steps that you can take to reduce any theoretical risk will also result in better-tasting coffee. Provided you don't drink too much of it (and there is no evidence of damage resulting from fewer than five cups a day), and don't boil it, you should come to no harm. There seems to be no good reason to believe that decaffeinated coffee is any better for you either, although you may prefer to reduce the stimulant effect associated with caffeine. If you are taking any homoeopathic remedies you should know that coffee is likely to antidote the remedy. It is not the caffeine which is significant here but the coffee itself, so you should abstain during the length of your treatment. Otherwise, it really is up to you. If coffee is your preferred drug of solace, there is nothing to suggest that drinking it in moderation will harm you.

Conclusions on substance use

Although social attitudes to them vary enormously, alcohol, tobacco and street drugs are all taken for similar reasons – to improve mood or to escape from intolerable emotional states or life circumstances. As such, lesbians taking refuge in the drugs of solace need to be aware that getting temporary relief from painful feelings is not a solution and may, indeed, make problems harder to deal with effectively. This is as true of prescription drugs such as tranquillizers or anti-depressants as it is of heroin. Getting support from friends or a counsellor, or making life changes, may offer much more long-lasting rewards. However, you could be in therapy five days a week for fifty years and not change the racism, homophobia and other *social* factors which may make life feel unbearable, and it is these wider social factors which have been implicated as the major cause of higher rates of alcoholism, drug abuse and suicide among lesbians.[13] This means that we all have to develop healthy ways of combating the stresses which confront us as we live our lives as lesbians.

Alternatives to drugs: combating stress

Stress is an inevitable and useful part of our lives. Without a certain amount of stress we could not function properly. However, stress overload is damaging. It can result in distressing and unpleasant symptoms and, in the long term, can damage health. Whatever stresses women confront in our daily lives – institutional or personal racism, poverty, childcare responsibilities, ageing, sexual harassment or violence, surviving childhood sexual abuse, unemployment, etc., etc. – living as a lesbian in a society which devalues and discriminates against us is an additional stress factor. At certain times in some lesbians' lives homophobia can lead to periods of extreme and traumatic stress, such as when fighting for custody of a child, being ousted from a job or your home because you are a lesbian, or going through the death of a partner or the end of a relationship. At such times, when most heterosexual people can expect sympathetic support, we may have to deal with our situation in isolation or even secrecy. So it is very important to develop strategies to deal with the effects of stress. Different approaches work for different women, and it is important to find what works for you so that you have something to call on when your stress load starts to get out of hand.

Sometimes we don't even recognize that we are feeling the effects of stress until very late. Many people don't start taking any steps to learn stress-calming techniques until they are in great distress and the matter has become urgent. It is very valuable to learn to recognize your own pattern of response to stress, to learn which stressors you are especially vulnerable to and to learn what works to defuse the effects of stress for you *before* you are facing a life crisis! Early signs that you are under stress may include:

- sleep difficulties – difficulty in getting to sleep, waking frequently during the night or waking very early in the morning and not being able to get back to sleep

- low energy or chronic feelings of fatigue and exhaustion

- irritability, moodiness, lack of concentration, forgetfulness, depression, emotional numbness, lack of interest in sex or apathy

- general aches and pains, headaches, muscle stiffness, pains in the neck, shoulder, chest or lower back

- indigestion, heartburn, diarrhoea or constipation, a faint feeling of nausea all the time, reduced appetite or increased need to binge (resulting in unusual increase or decrease in weight).

Any of these signs should alert us to the need to start seriously chilling out. If you ignore them, or take no steps to start looking after yourself, then you may find you start to get major sleep difficulties, stomach cramps, panic attacks or dizziness. Sometimes the physical signs that we are under stress may in themselves be frightening. Your blood pressure may increase and you may start to get odd sensations connected to your heartbeat or your breathing. You may feel that you cannot breathe properly, you may experience palpitations (a fluttering and rapid heartbeat for a few seconds), or your heart may appear to miss a beat and then thump wildly. These are scary, but are *not* usually an indication that something is seriously wrong with your heart. Palpitations and other strange heartbeat sensations can usually be calmed by taking a deep breath, holding it for a count of three and letting it out slowly. You may want to consult your doctor or health adviser to reassure yourself that there is nothing physically wrong with your heart, but you may find that beginning stress-reduction strategies stops the worrying symptoms in a few days or weeks.

Stress-calming techniques

There are many ways of reducing the effects of stress on the body. None of them will sort out your life and solve your problems – that remains to be done – but they will help you recover from stress and become strong enough and calm enough to deal with your life. Activities which help to relax and calm you, and to soothe that awful wound-up feeling include the following.

- *Take vigorous exercise.* This is the best of all, since it is the way in which our bodies are designed to eliminate adrenaline, the 'flight or fight' hormone which gives rise to stress symptoms. People who exercise regularly are better able to cope with stress, and those of us who are suffering from burn-out or stress overload find that it helps relaxation and improves sleep.

- *Take gentle exercise such as yoga, tai chi or swimming.* Yoga and tai chi can be especially beneficial, since they have developed over centuries to achieve states of inner peace and calm (oh yes!).

- *Take simple steps to regain a feeling of control in your life.* Talk to a counsellor, phone a helpline or get a therapist. Make a list of the things you feel stressed out by and see if you can let some of them go. Get professional help dealing with money or job problems; indeed, ask for help wherever and from whomever you can.

- *Increase the amount of pleasure in your life*, even if you don't feel as if you can enjoy anything. Part of you will be enjoying it, even if it doesn't feel like it! Get some favourite light reading out of your local library, have a friend round to watch a video or to go for a walk with in the country.

- *Try to reduce your intake of alcohol and tobacco and especially caffeine.* It took me two years of panic attacks to work out that they were caused by drinking more coffee each day than I could tolerate. Reducing your intake of coffee can help dramatically, but if you are a heavy coffee drinker you should not give it up suddenly, since you will get withdrawal symptoms. Reduce gradually, and aim for one cup a day, as a special treat.

- *Try to get looked after.* Treat yourself to a massage, or ask a friend to give you one. Try getting support from a complementary health practitioner (see below, Chapter 9). Acupuncture, homoeopathy, aromatherapy and hypnotherapy may all be able to reduce stress and help your body recover.

- *Be kind to your body.* Get plenty of rest (not necessarily sleep), luxuriate in long baths or slob about listening to your favourite music, massage foot lotion into your feet and legs, eat some favourite food.

You may feel that your stress level is making you really ill. If this is the case, have a look at the section on emotional health in Chapter 5.

Conclusion:
basic maintenance for dykes

We are all surviving in an environment which is basically health-damaging in many ways. You have only to count the number of adverts for herbal tranquillizers, calming New-Age music, relaxation therapies and stress-reduction handbooks to realize that being stressed out has become the norm for many millions of people. As lesbians, we have to deal with additional factors which compound or add to the damaging effects of contemporary life. Maintaining good health helps us stay fit and strong and more able to live well and happily as lesbians. It won't change the world but, if you want to change the world, looking after yourself will make you better able to do it.

Further reading

New books on healthy eating and exercise are constantly being published, and you are recommended to browse the shelves of your local bookshop. Books of special interest to lesbians, which include detailed advice on maintaining basic health, include *The New Our Bodies Ourselves*, and *Alive and Well* (see Chapter 1, Further reading for details). For older lesbians, there is much useful information in *Ourselves, Growing Older: Women Ageing with Knowledge and Power*, written by Paula Brown Doress and Diana Laskin Siegal in co-operation with the Boston Women's Health Book Collective (British edition by Jean Shapiro) and published in 1989 by Fontana, London.

Networking

Britain

For information about additives and organic foods:

The Soil Association, 86 Colston Street, Bristol BS1 5BB

For information and advice about vegetarianism/veganism:

Vegan Society, 33–5 George Street, Oxford OX1 2AY

Vegetarian Society, Parkdale, Dunham Road, Altrincham, Cheshire WA14 4QG

For general advice on food and nutrition:

The Women's Nutritional Advisory Service (WNAS), PO Box 268, Brighton, East Sussex BN3 1RW

For support and advice about alcohol:

Alcohol Concern, 305 Gray's Inn Road, London WC1X 8QF

Alcoholics Anonymous, PO Box 1, Stonebow House, Stonebow, York YO1 2NJ

Women's Alcohol Centre, 254 St Paul's Road, London N1 2LJ

For support and advice about street drugs:

RELEASE, 169 Commercial Street, London E1 6BW (emergency tel.: 0171-603-8654)

Narcotics Anonymous, PO Box 417, London SW10 0RN

For support and advice on eating disorders:

Anorexia and Bulimia Nervosa Association (ABNA), Tottenham Women's Health Centre, Annexe C, Tottenham Town Hall, London N5 4RX

USA

A comprehensive directory of the many services on offer can be obtained from the National Lesbian and Gay Health Foundation Inc., PO Box 65472, Washington DC 20035.

Canada

Lesbian Health Guide, edited by Regan McClure and Anne Vespry and published by Queer Press, Toronto, 1994, contains detailed information about maintaining good health, together with an extensive directory of organizations and further reading.

Australia and New Zealand

The New Our Bodies Ourselves contains an extensive directory of services, groups and newsletters in New Zealand and all the territories of Australia.

3 Playing Safe, Playing Healthy: Sexual Health

There are many myths about lesbian sexual activity and almost as many about the health risks of sex between women. This section explodes some of the more common myths, and gives you the information you need to enjoy a safe, healthy and happy sex life. If you're not sure about the exact meaning of some of the words used, check them out on the diagram below.

What are the health risks in sex between women?

Sexual activity between women can pose two main kinds of risk. First, there is the risk of infection. There are many infections which may be transmitted sexually, some of which are merely unpleasant but a few of which can result in serious damage to your health. Some may even be life-threatening. Second, some sexual activities carry a risk of physical injury to one or both partners. It is better to predict such risks beforehand, so that they can be avoided, rather than ruin a tender moment by an embarrassing and painful visit to the accident and emergency department of your local hospital.

But I thought lesbians were safe from STDs?

As a group, lesbians tend to have a very low incidence of sexually transmitted diseases (STDs). For this reason, it is reasonable to think of lesbian sexual activity as 'safer' than most. However, low risk is

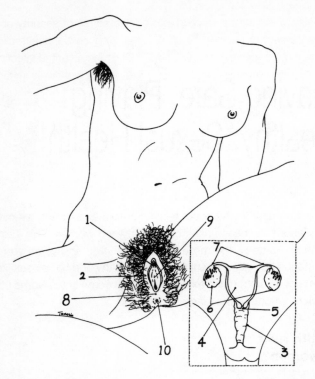

1 *Clitoris*. The only organ in the human body with no other function than sexual pleasure.

2 *Vulva*. The inner and outer lips of the vulva are called the labia.

3 *Vagina*. Strong, muscular channel capable of contracting powerfully in orgasm or childbirth.

4 *Uterus/womb*. Small muscular chamber which, in women of childbearing age, grows and sheds a new lining every month or so.

5 *Cervix*. The 'neck' of the womb, with a tiny hole in the middle (the os). It is this part of the womb which is affected by cervical cancer, and from which cells are scraped when you have a 'smear test'.

6 *Ovaries*. Walnut sized and shaped, these complex little organs store and regularly release eggs the size of a full stop. They also produce hormones which regulate the monthly cycle. A newborn baby girl's ovaries already contain all the eggs she will release in her lifetime.

7 *Fallopian tubes*. They have tiny fronds which draw each egg down into the womb to await fertilization (or your next period).

8 *Perineum*. Area between the vagina and the anus.

9 *Urethra*. Channel through which urine passes from the bladder.

10 *Anus*: The anal sphincter is a ring of strong muscle at the entrance to the rectum.

not no risk, and some lesbian health care workers are concerned that lesbians have been lulled into a false sense of security about STDs. Recent studies with lesbians attending sexual health clinics in London found that a significant number of them carried infections, including herpes and human pappilomavirus (a wart virus linked to cervical cancer).

Prevention: the first steps

Sexually transmitted infections are miserable and can be serious. Prevention is much better than cure, and a little care will help ensure that you avoid infection altogether or spot possible infections before they have a chance to do serious damage. Take your sexual health seriously! It is often the case that heterosexual women pay far more attention to cyclical changes in their bodies than lesbian women do, simply because pregnancy tends to be a more immediate concern. But an awareness of your cycles is important to help you recognize changes which may be early warning signs. One advantage that lesbians have over heterosexual women is that we tend to have more first-hand knowledge about women's bodies, and are more comfortable with female sexuality. Take advantage of this. Get to know your body intimately; how it looks, smells, tastes, feels. Pay loving attention to the body of anyone you have sex with, not to turn passion into suspicion or hypochondria but to help safeguard gorgeous lesbian bodies from ill health.

HIV/AIDS: should we ditch the latex?

Human Immunodeficiency Virus (HIV) is the infection most closely associated with the practice of safer sex. There is good reason to believe that HIV has been around since the mid- to late-1950s, although it was recognized by the medical profession only in the early 1980s in the USA. This is a virus which poses unique problems for prevention and cure. Viruses are the smallest living thing we know of, and are not capable of independent existence. HIV replicates by breaking into human white blood cells, the 'T-helper' cells, where it makes use of the cell's genetic material to reproduce itself. As it multiplies it eventually kills off the host cell and breaks out into the bloodstream to infect others. Eventually, it kills off T-cells faster than the body can replace them. The T-cells co-ordinate the body's complex immune response and, as the number of T-cells declines, so the immune system begins to break down, leaving the body vulnerable to a wide range of *opportunistic infections*. There are over a hundred of such infections now associated with HIV-related immune damage. They are caused by bacteria, viruses, protozoa and fungi and range from the commonplace (such as candida or thrush, which can be extremely unpleasant for someone with HIV) to diseases which, before the advent of this epidemic, were extremely rare – such as Kaposi's Sarcoma (KS), a form of skin cancer, or Pneumocystic Carinii Pneumonia (PCP), a previously rare form of pneumonia. At the stage where someone with HIV infection begins to develop recognized opportunistic infections, and their T-cell count falls below a certain level, they are said to have AIDS (Acquired Immune Deficiency Syndrome). AIDS is not a disease, it is a condition of drastically weakened immune response. It is not AIDS that eventually results in death, but one or more of the opportunistic infections, although HIV infection *itself* can also cause serious damage to the brain and central nervous system.

Taking an HIV test

If you have reason to suspect that you may be infected with HIV, you should go to your local Genito-Urinary Medicine (GUM) clinic, where you will receive counselling and informed advice about whether or not to take a test. If you do decide to be tested, a small sample of your blood will be taken and tested for antibodies to HIV. The results of this test, however, are not necessarily conclusive. Normally the body responds to infections by producing *antibodies* to begin fighting the invading organism. For reasons as yet poorly understood this process may be very much delayed in people newly infected with HIV. Antibodies may not appear for several weeks, or even many months, after infection. This means that they may not show up on an antibody test, which is the main way of ascertaining whether or not someone has HIV. If you take an antibody test and it is negative you may be asked to come back for a second test several weeks later, and to avoid any activities which may result in infection in the meantime. People whose antibody test gives a positive result (and this may be confirmed by using another test) are said to be 'HIV-positive' or to have 'sero-converted'.

When antibodies do appear, they are ineffective against this new virus. No doubt our bodies are evolving an immune response to HIV, but this process takes many generations and will not take effect in our lifetime. The virus also has an extremely long incubation period. It may remain in the body for many years before symptoms are noticed. Some people have a brief flu-like illness around the time that they become infected, but this is not true for everyone, and many people simply interpret this 'acute HIV infection' as a cold or flu. Some people may develop persistant swollen glands in the groin, armpit and neck (PGL), or have drenching night sweats, but this too is not the case for everyone. The long symptom-free period is excellent news for people who have HIV, but it represents an enormous problem for controlling the epidemic. It makes it very hard to get an accurate idea of the number of people infected, and means that most people who are infected probably do not know.

Staying uninfected

The virus also appears capable of very rapid alterations to its outer 'shell'. It is this shell that must be 'recognized' if a vaccine is to be effective, and the fact that HIV can change its shell many times during its residence in one individual poses a very serious problem for the development of a vaccine. Even if a vaccine were to be developed, the cost of vaccinating sufficient numbers of people to make a perceptible impact on the spread of the epidemic would be astronomical – enough to bankrupt any developing nation and well out of the reach of many developed nations.

There is no vaccine or cure for HIV infection, and the eventual outcome is an immune system so badly damaged that survival is not possible. The good news is that it is not easy to catch; the only way to get HIV from someone who is infected is if you share street drug injecting equipment or have unsafe sex with them. An HIV-positive mother may pass the virus on to her child during pregnancy or birth (breastfeeding represents a low risk). So safer sex and drug use are important in preventing transmission. There is also the important point that sexual practices which prevent the transmission of HIV will also prevent the transmission of most other STDs. But information about HIV in lesbian communities is confusing. While some community activists insist that we should all buy the safe sex videos, stock up on dental dams and lubricants and learn how to practise safer sex, others declare that sex between women *is* safe sex, that dental dams and latex gloves are unnecessary, and that lesbians shouldn't be panicked into restricting their sexual relationships with women in any way.

It is important to approach the idea of 'risk' in a thoughtful way. It is certainly the case that there have been very few recorded cases of woman-to-woman transmission of HIV. The number of such cases is tiny, and, in such cases as there are, the route of transmission is generally disputed. However, there *are* substantial numbers of lesbians with HIV, and there are lesbians working in AIDS service organizations who are convinced that transmission between women is possible. If you are HIV-positive, learning about safer sex will not only offer protection to your sexual partners, but will also help you to avoid infection with other bacteria, viruses and fungi which can be serious for someone with HIV-compromised immunity. If you are currently HIV-negative you should assume at the very least that there may be a time when you are lovers with a woman who is HIV-positive. She should not have to teach you about safer sex (she may not have adequate information herself in any case), and you will need to know

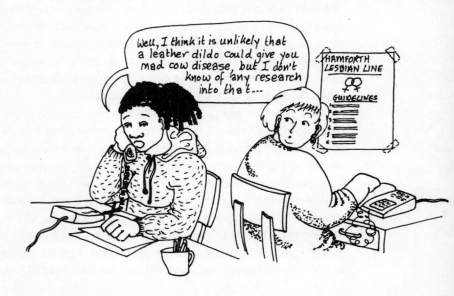

not only how to prevent transmission of HIV between you but also how to protect her from other infections which may put her health at risk.

There are problems with the collection of official data about lesbians and HIV. For example, the Center for Disease Control, the body which monitors the epidemic in the United States, will record a woman as a lesbian only if she has had sex *exclusively* with women since 1977. Additionally, many lesbians have good reason not to risk making their sexuality known to medical staff, so there is likely to be an under-reporting of HIV infection among lesbians. It is also probably true that lesbians who know they have HIV are likely to attribute their infection to previous sexual activity with men or to injecting drug use, since it is so widely believed that lesbian sex is 'safe'.

Despite all these reasons to distrust the figures, it remains the case that the sexual transmission of HIV between women is rare. A recent study reported in *The Lancet* concluded that 'Our results support a non-existent risk of viral transmission in HIV-discordant lesbian couples engaging in sex acts that have a theoretically high transmission risk'. In other words, when one woman is known to have HIV and the other is known not to, the risk of transmission between them during sex appears 'non-existent'. However, it is important to bear in mind that this research was done on a small sample – just eighteen couples.

Unfortunately, nobody is in a position to be able to say categorically that HIV transmission during sex between women is impossible. We can safely conclude that it is *rare*. But physical risk is not the only concern. Lesbians who know they have HIV, their partners and any lesbian who is anxious and fearful about the virus, need to know how to have sex in a way which feels *safe enough for them*. It makes sense to inform yourself about safer sex, but you will need to make your own decision about when and where *you* feel you need to use it.

Staying safe

HIV is incapable of living outside the body, and can infect you only by getting into your bloodstream. The theoretical risks in sex between two women are in any activity where an HIV-positive woman's blood (including menstrual blood) or juices from her vagina can enter the bloodstream of her partner. This is possible only through recently damaged skin or mucus membrane, such as the soft tissues lining the mouth, vagina or anus.

There has been an assumption in the AIDS literature that the only thing lesbians do is cunnilingus, which is why dental dams have been promoted as safer sex for lesbians. Dams are squares of latex which may be used as a barrier between your tongue and her body (or vice versa) in order to prevent menstrual blood or vaginal juices coming into contact with the mucus membrane of the mouth. If cunnilingus was high-risk, dams would be promoted in safer sex campaigns aimed at straights. They are not, and cunnilingus is generally regarded as low-risk. There is a *theoretical* risk that the virus may be transmitted this way and, if one of you knows or suspects that she might have HIV, you may wish to consider using a dam. It will also help prevent you passing other infections, such as herpes, thrush and hepatitis. *This* is important, especially for women who are HIV-positive, since other infections may be particularly unpleasant and dangerous for them. We should think of HIV-positive lesbians as vulnerable, not dangerous, and as being at risk from their HIV-negative sisters rather than the other way around.

How to use a latex barrier

If you cannot get hold of dental dams, or if you find them too thick, use a condom instead. Unroll the condom, carefully cut the top off with *sharp* scissors and cut it open along its length. Open it out, wash off the lubricant (which tastes foul) and you have a barrier which can be used for oral sex. A little lubricant spread on the area to be licked will add to the pleasure and prevent the possibility of sticking. Gently spread the lips of her vulva and stretch the latex tightly over it with your hands. You can work it into place around her clit with your lips and tongue. It is tricky at first, but gets much easier with practice. Remember that the whole point is to keep your mouth and her juices separate, so don't reuse cut-up condoms (dams are thicker and can be washed in warm soapy water, rinsed, and patted dry) and don't get the two sides mixed up. Remember, oil-based lubricants (Vaseline, baby oil, massage oils) will destroy the latex.

And don't use talcum powder to dry dams, it is linked to ovarian cancer.

It is difficult to imagine how any other lesbian sexual activity could result in effective transmission of HIV. Things that may cause bruising or bleeding to the vagina or rectum, such as fisting, or vigorous fucking with fingers, dildos or sex toys, are possibly a risk if the damaged tissues are then exposed to contact with semen or with your partner's blood. If you play with men remember that semen can contain large quantities of virus and should *not* come into contact with your vagina or anus, or with any recent cuts. The possibility of infection through cuts or sores on your hands is negligible, but if you are concerned, use disposable latex gloves for finger-fucking or fisting, and use plenty of lubricant.

Condom use for lesbians: other STDs

Other STDs are more infectious than HIV, so it is a sensible precaution to use condoms on dildos or other toys, and to change the condom between users. I don't want to suggest you leap into bed with vet's calving gloves on (unless it turns you on), but if you are finger-fucking her and yourself, remember that it is possible to pass infections from one to another with those lovely sticky fingers. Perhaps your right hand for her, your left hand for you? Think about it. It is especially important not to put anything which has been in your or her anus into anyone's vagina, since bacteria and other micro-organisms which flourish happily and harmlessly in the rectum can be extremely unpleasant if they get into the vagina or urethra. Nobody is suggesting that you have to stop having sex with bare hands, but if you enjoy penetration and one of you knows or suspects that she has an infection of some kind, you can use condoms (over two fingers, dildo or whatever) and lubricant. Don't move your hand or fingers from anus to vagina without washing with hot soapy water. Yes, it's a drag but not half as much of a drag as having to give up sex for weeks and limp around dripping antibiotic pessaries, live yoghurt or garlic, trying to get rid of some miserable infection. Take it from one who knows!

Some STDs to look out for

Not every possible STD is on this list, so check the resources section for more information. If you suspect that you may have an infection please *don't* wait for it to get better or go away. Symptoms may indeed disappear, but unfortunately this doesn't always mean that the infection has gone away. Many serious STDs can hang around undetected for a very long time (HIV, gonorrhoea and syphilis for example), and can cause permanent damage.

Thrush

Also called candida, this is a common fungal infection. The fungus lives naturally in the moist, warm conditions of the vagina, where it is kept at bay by the natural acidity of vaginal secretions. Any change in the levels of acidity can give rise to an attack, and this can be linked to stress, change in diet or a course of antibiotics. Symptoms are a thick, curd-like discharge with a not unpleasant yeasty smell and an intolerable itching and burning sensation in the genital area. Some women treat it successfully by applying live yoghurt or garlic, but it is important to get a proper diagnosis, since there are other infections which can mimic some of the symptoms. If you go to a GUM clinic, they will take a swab from your vagina; if you go to your GP you should insist on this being done. There are effective treatments available, and it is probably a good idea to get your partner checked for infection too, since it is possible to reinfect each other. It is especially important for HIV-positive women to avoid outbreaks of thrush where possible, since it is a stubborn and invasive condition when associated with HIV-related damage to the immune system.

Chlamydia

It used to be thought that this was a relatively minor infection, but we now know that it can have serious consequences. In women it can lead to Pelvic Inflammatory Disease (PID), an extremely unpleasant and hard-to-treat condition, and (for dykes trying to get pregnant) it has been linked to post-abortion complications, ectopic pregnancy (pregnancy in the fallopian.tubes) and miscarriage.

Symptoms may include thin vaginal discharge, low abdominal pain and fever, but they may be so mild as to pass unnoticed. It is not known whether sex between women can transmit chlamydia, but it is by far the commonest form of STD, so it seems likely that it can. Diagnosis requires specialist laboratory equipment and taking a swab from the cervix. In men, chlamydia is often refered to as 'NSU', so if you have ever had a male partner with this diagnosis (or if you have ever had a diagnosis of NSU yourself) it may be worth getting tested.

Syphilis

This used to be a great epidemic killer; now it is treatable with antibiotics and is no longer a common infection in the industrialized nations. It is spread by a bacterium and the first symptom is usually a small, painless sore (a 'chancre') on or near the genitals, mouth, anus or even the breast or fingertips. It may develop inside the mouth, anus or vagina, where it goes unnoticed, and most women with syphilis do not recognize it. The chancre is the point of entry of the disease into the body, and it is highly infectious while it lasts. It disappears in a few weeks, but the bacteria then spread throughout the body, causing rashes, sores in the mouth, painful joints or aching bones, sore throat, headache or mild fever. Such symptoms come and go during this 'secondary' stage. The disease then becomes 'latent', giving no outward symptoms, but progressing through internal organs; finally, at the 'late' stage, severe damage done to internal organs results in death, blindness, mental confusion or paralysis. It is very rare nowadays for the disease to progress to the final stage and it is diagnosed by a simple blood test, which is routine at all GUM clinics. Pregnant women are also routinely tested for syphilis, since it can harm the unborn infant.

Gonorrhoea

This bacterial infection can affect the cervix, urethra, anus and throat and may be transmitted from one woman to another on fingers or a dildo or through oral sex. It is a difficult infection to spot, since early symptoms are very mild. Around half of women with gonorrhoea fail to recognize the infection until it is picked up by clinical tests. If untreated, infection can lead to Pelvic Inflammatory Disease (which is painful and serious). If allowed to spread it may infect other organs throughout the body, resulting in blindness, damage to the heart or arthritic meningitis. Treatment with antibiotics is effective, so serious damage is now rare in industrialized countries.

Symptoms usually appear between two days and a few weeks after infection. You may notice an unusual discharge from your vagina or rectum, pain on urination or painful bowel movements. If the infection spreads up into the body, you may have pain on one or both sides of your lower abdomen, with vomiting and fever. Periods may become irregular. A swab taken from the infected part will be cultured, and a course of antibiotics prescribed.

Herpes

Before the advent of HIV, herpes was the recurring nightmare of the sexually adventurous. It is spread by the herpes simplex virus, and causes acutely painful sores around the mouth, anus or genitals. It can also affect the eyes – one good reason why contact lens wearers should take care to wash their hands when inserting or removing lenses. It can be transmitted by oral sex. Once infected, you are infected for life. This does not mean you will be plastered with painful sores for ever: symptoms come and go and, although many factors can trigger a fresh outbreak (stress, other illness, pregnancy etc.), the first outbreak is usually the worst.

Around half of all adults have herpes antibodies in their blood (which indicates that they have been exposed to the virus), yet only a few ever suffer from recurrent attacks. Individuals have very different experiences of herpes and it can be maddeningly unpleasant. There are two types of the virus, HSVI and HSVII. The first is generally responsible for cold sores around the mouth, the second for painful sores around the genitals or anus. Herpes can be particularly unpleasant in people with HIV infection: if you or your partner are HIV-positive, this is one extra infection to guard against carefully.

Symptoms begin with an itching or tingling sensation in the affected area and then sores begin to appear. Initially these are red bumps but within a day or so they develop into watery blisters. There may also be a burning sensation or pain in the legs, buttocks or genitals, accompanied by a feeling of pressure. The blisters burst, leaving shallow ulcers which weep and bleed, and finally form scabs and heal. Sometimes there is a fever, swollen glands or headache. The first outbreak generally takes between two and six weeks to clear up, and the sores are highly infectious during this time. Effective treatment is difficult: this is one infection to avoid if at all possible! During symptom-free periods the chance of acquiring herpes from an infected person are remote, so the golden rule is to avoid contact with any rashes or sores which you suspect might be due to herpes, and get a diagnosis confirmed as soon as possible.

If you are diagnosed with herpes it can have a serious effect on your sex life, so it is important to get support. Contact a self-help group (ask at your GUM clinic for information) or the Herpes Association for up-to-date information about treatments. You are likely to find that advice assumes heterosexuality; lesbians are less likely than straight women to have herpes, so if you want to talk to other lesbians with herpes you may have to start you own local support group. If you have herpes, you are infectious during an outbreak. At this time you should not allow anyone to lick or kiss your genitals, and you and your partner(s) should take great care during sex not to pass on the infection.

Genital warts

These are not a problem in themselves, but there is a strong link between the wart virus (Human Papilloma Virus: HPV) and cervical cancer. It used to be believed that cervical cancer was a problem only for women who have sex with men, but recent studies show that this is probably not the case. Although there is good evidence that penile penetration (especially without a condom) is a high-risk activity for cervical cancer, it is not the only risk. Regular smears (see pp. 206–8) are important for lesbians too.

Early symptoms of wart virus infection take from a few weeks to a few months to appear. Small, painless hard spots appear, usually at the bottom of the opening to the vagina. They may also occur inside the vagina, on the labia or the cervix or around the anus. Laser treatment is now the preferred way of eliminating genital warts, though it is possible to burn them off with caustic chemical solutions as well. *Don't attempt to do this yourself using over-the-counter wart treatments.*

The wart virus may be passed during sex between women, on hands or sex toys. Don't worry about conventional warts on the hands or fingers: these are caused by a different virus.

Parasites

It is also possible to pass tiny parasitic insects from one woman to another during sex. These include *crabs* (lice that live on pubic hair) and *scabies* (tiny mites that burrow beneath the skin). Both are spread by direct skin contact with the infected area. Scabies may not cause any symptoms for the first few days, so it is possible to pass it on to a partner before you know you've got it. Crabs cause itching in the genital area, and you may be able to see the insects or their eggs around your pubic hair. They are killed using chemicals, and you will need to treat all members of your household and recent sex partners to prevent recurring infestation. Wash all bedding and underwear. If you are unlucky enough to get crabs, try not to scratch, since this can cause infection.

Scabies causes intense itching and raised, red weals or bumps on the skin. They may be found in folds in the skin, on the hands, between the fingers, around the genitals, buttocks or under the breasts. Again, don't scratch, since the infection caused by scratching is often worse than the original condition. It can be hard to diagnose, since it may be confused with allergies, eczema and other skin problems. A small scraping from the affected area needs to be examined under a microscope for a firm diagnosis. Make sure your doctor does this, as the chemicals used to treat scabies are toxic, and shouldn't be applied unless you know they are needed.

Bacterial vaginosis

This has been found to be the commonest sexually transmissible infection among lesbians. It is not one infection but several, and the name simply refers to an infection of the vagina caused by a bacterium. The commonest causes a watery, slightly fishy-smelling discharge, and is sometimes associated with a bacterium called gardnerella. You can certainly pass these bacterial infections during woman-to-woman sex, so any discharge, itching or discomfort should be checked out at your GUM clinic. There is a high recurrence rate for bacterial vaginosis, so it is a good idea to take your partner along and get her treated as well, so that you do not continually reinfect each other. You will be prescribed tablets or pessaries (to be inserted into the vagina), and it is important that you follow the instructions and finish the course, to prevent the bacteria developing resistance. If you have to use pessaries, you can prevent them staining your knickers by using sanitary towels.

How to stay sexy and healthy

STDs are less common among lesbians than among other sexually active groups in the population, but we do get them and we can pass them on to each other when having sex. Follow a few golden rules to reduce the risk to yourself and your partners, and to make sure you spot any potential problem before it gets to be serious.

Golden rules for a healthy sex life

- Find out how to play safely – learn safer sex techniques and be sensible about putting them into practice.

- Take care of your body. Look out for any discharge from vagina, urethra or anus which is unusual for you, and get it checked out.

- If you feel pain when you use the toilet or during sex, get it checked out.

- Any unusual or unexplained pain in the lower abdomen, whether on one side or on both, should be checked out.

- Any unusual bleeding from the anus or vagina needs to be checked out.

- Have regular smear tests and once in a while get a thorough sexual health check-up.

- Eat well, sleep well, be sensible around alcohol and recreational drugs, don't smoke.

- Get to know your partner's body as well as you know your own.

- If you or your partner has HIV, any other immune disorder, reduced sensation in your genital area, incontinence problems or mobility restrictions, take extra care to avoid STD infection.

Do you always hurt the one you love?

As well as the risk of infection, some sexual practices carry their own risk of injury. With a little thought, you can avoid accidentally hurting the one you love, whether the kind of sex you enjoy is sadomasochistic or 'vanilla'.

Sadomasochism (S/M) covers a wide range of sex play, from highly ritualized 'scenes' making use of purpose-built dungeons and expensive equipment to less specialized games which many people would not consider S/M at all. There is no rigid division between S/M and vanilla sex, and no guarantee that either will make you more politically aware, exciting, grown-up or sexy. Inequalities of power are present in sexual exchanges whether we like it or not, and issues of consent, abuse and violence are important questions in *all* lesbian relationships, not just those between self-identified sadomasochists. Whatever kind of sex you like, you need to consider both the physical and the emotional safety of yourself and your partner.

There are guidelines and informal rules which the S/M community has established to try and ensure the safety of its members. If you are into S/M, do read Pat Califia's safety guide, *The Lesbian S/M Safety Manual*. Some feminist and community bookshops in Britain refuse to stock it; if you have trouble getting hold of a copy then Gay's The Word bookshop in London will send you one (see Further reading, below). The key do's and don'ts are as follows, and *many of them are as important in 'vanilla' sex as they are in S/M*. Just because you don't handcuff your partner doesn't mean sex between you is never going to be emotionally risky.

- Do agree limits and safe words with your partner *before you start*. For example, what you like and don't like, what you are and are not prepared to do. This is not just a good idea for S/M players.

- Do stick to any agreements you make about what kinds of sex you both like. Don't break them in the heat of the moment.

- Do attend to emotional safety: be prepared to handle tears, shaking or (especially) any traumatic memories of past abuse which may surface during a 'scene'. This may happen to women who have been abused in the past, whether or not the sex they are having is S/M.

- Do develop strategies for reassuring and calming a partner who becomes distressed: the old-fashioned cup of tea and a cuddle can be very effective, but some women prefer *not* to be held if, for example, memories of abuse surface. Check it out.

- Do learn from experience with a partner. If something has caused her distress in the past, don't play games with it.

- Don't use alcohol or drugs when doing S/M. Both weaken concentration and judgement and may make it much harder to take care of each other.

- Do have basic first-aid equipment on hand if you are doing anything which is likely to result in burning or bleeding, and know how to use it.

- Don't flap about like a headless chicken if something seems to be seriously wrong. If in doubt, get to the accident and emergency department of your local hospital. They've seen it all before, and dealing with strange looks is much better than dealing with possibly dangerous injuries.

- Don't play around with suffocation ('breath control'); it's too dangerous, since even a few seconds without oxygen can cause permanent brain damage.

- Don't improvise bondage out of silk scarves, ropes, wires, etc. They can all cause nerve damage if they pull too tightly for too long, and all can be very difficult to release in an emergency. Use proper leather cuffs from a supplier, and fit panic bolts for quick release. For spur-of-the-moment light bondage, keep scissors at hand in case you have to cut her free.

- Don't ignore any of the following during or after an S/M scene, they all require medical attention:
  - loss of consciousness for more than a second or two
  - confusion or blurred speech/vision
  - bleeding from vagina or anus
  - cuts, weals or bruises which become red, inflamed and hot and/or weep

- fever, lethargy or confusion a day or two after anal fisting – this could indicate peritonitis, which is potentially fatal

- vomiting, and/or dull, aching pain in the abdomen, or sudden onset of severe abdominal pain

- difficulty breathing (asthmatics should always have an inhaler to hand and both of you should know how to use it)

- Don't let excitement or your need to prove something make you go beyond the limits of either of you, physically or emotionally.

> Whether the kind of sex we enjoy is something we are happy to call S/M or not, it makes sense to look after ourselves and our lovers. What follows is a run-down of some things which lesbians like to do, together with hints on how to minimize the possible risks of infection or injury. Remember that lesbian sex is generally *very safe*: this list is intended to give you the information you need to reduce any risks to the absolute minimum. Please don't think you have to approach sex scrubbed and gloved like a surgeon, you don't!

- *Cunnilingus* (licking or kissing or sucking the clitoris and labia). This is low-risk in terms of HIV, although it can transmit herpes and other STDs such as syphilis, gonorrhoea and chlamydia. You can use a dental dam or a cut-up condom between licker and licked (see p. 60) if you are concerned.

- *Rimming* (licking or tonguing the anus). This is low-risk in terms of HIV infection and possible injury, but carries a risk of bacterial, amoebal and parasitic infections. Wash the anus beforehand with soap and water (enemas are not necessary), and use a dam or a cut-up condom as a barrier between licker and licked if you want to reduce the risk of infection (see p. 60).

- *Finger-fucking* (inserting a finger or fingers into the vagina or anus). Low-risk in terms of infection or physical damage. Make sure hands are clean and nails are short and smooth, with no jagged edges or hang nails to cause painful scratches. *Never* force anything into the vagina or anus, and *never* move anything (including fingers) from anus to vagina without washing in between. If you are especially worried about infection, perhaps because of fresh cuts or sores on your hands, you can use disposable latex gloves (from any chemist) or put a condom on a couple of fingers, though this is unlikely to be necessary.

- *Fisting* (inserting the entire hand into the vagina or anus). Low-risk for STDs but it is easy to cause physical harm, especially with anal fisting. Fisting needs to be done slowly (finger by finger), carefully and with plenty of lubricant, and nails must be kept short and smooth. It is possible to bruise the vagina, and women who have had an episiotomy (a surgical cut to enlarge the vagina during childbirth) may find it too painful. Care should be taken not to bruise the cervix or the urethra (see p. 54). Anal fisting can easily result in tears to the lining of the rectum, or to the lower bowel (which is fragile). This may cause peritonitis, if the contents of the bowel leak into the abdomenal cavity. Peritonitis is *serious* and can be rapidly fatal. *Seek medical help urgently for anyone who becomes feverish or lethargic after being fisted.* Unless you are very determined in your pursuit of anal pleasure, it is much easier and safer to stick to vaginal fisting.

- *Using a dildo or butt plug* to penetrate the vagina or anus is low-risk in terms of infection, provided the toys are not shared and are not passed from anus to vagina. If you plan to do either of these things, wash them with hot soapy water between users, or use a condom and change it between users. Leather toys cannot be washed and should *always* be used with a condom. It is possible to cause bruising by penetrating either vagina or anus with an inanimate object, especially if either of you has reduced sensation or awareness due to an impairment/injury or to alcohol or other drugs. If you are using a dildo in a harness, be aware that it is easy for it to slip out without you noticing and to bruise the one being fucked. Use with sensitivity – it is better (and often more pleasurable) not to withdraw completely when fucking. Take particular care with the anus, don't put anything very far in, and don't leave anything in there which could 'get lost'. Purpose-designed butt plugs, with flared ends, are the safest bet. If you do get anything stuck in your anus, don't try to poke it out, just sit on the toilet and see if you can get it to come out by gently bearing down. If not, off to casualty!

- *Watersports/golden showers* (playing with urine/piss). Low-risk in terms of STDs, but should not be used on broken skin or anywhere near eyes. If ingested, there is a risk from some infections, so drink your own, not hers.

- *Scat/choccie drops* (playing with faeces/shit). High-risk for a range of infections (though probably not HIV). Use latex gloves, don't let it get into your vagina, mouth or eyes, and keep away from broken skin. Follow the instructions carefully if using enemas, and avoid using them too often.

- *Piercings* should *always* be done by a reputable professional, since there is a risk of infection (including HIV infection) by cross-contamination. If you or your partner has a recent piercing, stick to the care instructions you have been given, and be sensible about your sexual practices. You may have had those rings put in your nipples or labia precisely in order to play with them during sex, but *do* wait until they have properly healed, or you risk infection and/or a nasty tear.

Getting seen to:
how to use sexual health services

It is important to have access to health care services that you trust and which are user-friendly. In the area of sexual health this is even more important. Many lesbians have had problems dealing with homophobic medical professionals, and there is a lot of ignorance concerning lesbian sexual health among health professionals as well as among lesbians themselves.

An important part of taking care of yourself as a lesbian is making sure that you can get regular cervical smears (see pp. 206–8) and health checks when you need them, and that you can get prompt, informed and effective treatment and care for any sexual health problems you may have. You are most likely to have all those needs met if you make use of specialist sexual health facilities. In Britain this means the genito-urinary medicine (GUM) clinics run by the NHS, rather than your general practitioner (GP). GPs are skilled generalists; they have to know how to diagnose an extraordinarily wide range of problems. Few of them are likely to have the specialist knowledge needed to spot some of the more subtle STDs, and even fewer will be able to offer advice which is based on a sound knowledge of lesbian sexual behaviour and health care needs. If you are lucky enough to have a lesbian GP, make use of her, but it is still probably a good idea to familiarize yourself with your local GUM clinic.

GUM clinics are listed in the phone book (some still under 'VD clinic'). They are run along lines of strict confidentiality, and you are at liberty to give a false name if you wish. They treat plenty of 'Jane Austen's! Depending on what exactly you have come into contact with you may be asked to help with 'contact tracing'. This involves informing other sexual partners that they may have been exposed to infection; this is an important way of controlling the spread of diseases such as gonorrhoea (efficient contact tracing is one reason why gonorrhoea has been so effectively controlled in Britain). Make it clear if you do not wish your identity to become known to the sexual partners involved, although this is not inevitable and GUM clinics are experienced in doing this without compromising their clients. It is in their interests to be sensitive and efficient, since they hope to encourage contact tracing as a means of infection control.

It is certainly the case that GUM clinics have the knowledge, experience and facilities (laboratory back-up, etc.) to make them the most likely source of accurate diagnosis and appropriate, effective treatment. They are also by far the best places to go if you need an HIV antibody test, since the test results will not be passed to your GP. You will obviously want to remain in control of who has access to information about your antibody status, and you need to plan carefully when to involve your GP in this. You are also most likely to receive informed counselling and advice before and after you take the test, and this includes advice about services and support.

Lesbian clinics

In an ideal world we would all be able to use GUM services run by lesbians for lesbians. The good news is that these are available in many cities in the USA and Canada, and are starting up in Britain. The Sandra Bernhardt and Audre Lorde clinics in London are specialist lesbian sexual health clinics, and have proved very popular among lesbians. Both Oxford and Glasgow now offer specialist lesbian sexual health clinics (see local gay press for details), and health authorities in other cities are interested in setting up similar clinics – your local lesbian and gay switchboard will have details of any near you. Lesbian sexual health clinics do not necessarily employ lesbian-only staff, but all staff are lesbian-friendly and informed about lesbian issues. They will all see women from outside their area but, if you intend to travel a long way, do ring up and see whether you need an appointment.

> 66 I got a letter from my doctor telling me that the results of my smear test were abnormal, and that I should go back for another test. I panicked, and couldn't bear the thought of going through the whole business again. So I got on the bus and went up to London for the day and booked myself in for a full sexual health check-up at the Bernhardt clinic. It was great! They were really friendly, explained everything very clearly, and seemed to have all the time in the world to answer my questions (including one about the warts on my girlfriend's fingers that I would never have had the guts to ask my doctor). The doctor was very respectful and gentle, and the tests were all done with great care. Best of all, the waiting room was full of cute lesbians! 99

'Elizabeth'

Complementary medicine

Alternative/complementary therapies are often useful in sexual health problems, especially those where conventional treatments are ineffective or have problematic side effects. However, it is unfair to expect most alternative practitioners to be able to diagnose specific infections without the kind of specialist equipment needed, and it is generally good advice to go to a clinic to get a diagnosis and *then* have a word with your homoeopath, acupuncturist, herbalist or other practitioner about treatments. Some complementary therapies may be very useful in preventing or minimizing the side-effects of strong drug treatments, such as powerful antibiotics, or in building up your general health after an infection.

Sex with men

If you have penetrative sex with men, please remember that it can make you pregnant, and that it is much easier to get a sexually transmitted infection from a man than it is from a woman. Always use a condom, with lubricant, and don't assume that this will be adequate protection against pregnancy. Any women's health handbook will give you advice about contraception but, unless you are contemplating a long-term sexual relationship with a man, it is best to avoid the pill or the IUD (coil) and stick to methods that have less impact on your health. These include the cap or vaginal condom. You will need to be fitted with a cap and taught how to use it. If you need advice about contraception, the best place to get it is a family planning clinic. Despite the off-puttingly heterosexual name, they are experienced, broad-minded and generally staffed by women. However, they are currently in the middle of a funding crisis, and you may have no alternative but to consult your regular doctor.

Of course, sex with men does not *have* to include penile penetration. You can stick to manual or oral sex, which will dramatically reduce your risk of pregnancy or infections. But remember that most straight men (and some gay men) don't regard it as 'real sex' unless they get to fuck you. Check this out beforehand. The power dynamic between men and women is very different to what goes on between women, and many men (gay and straight) are just not used to talking to women about sex. If you are unfamiliar with this, you may find it difficult to get your needs met.

If you have had unprotected sex with a man, whether with or without your consent, do find out about the 'morning-after pill', which can stop you becoming pregnant if taken soon enough after you had sex, and think carefully about whether you want an HIV test. Ring your GUM clinic for advice on both these points. You will probably have to get the morning-after pill from your doctor, but you may be able to get it from a family planning clinic or well woman clinic.

And finally . . .

Don't allow worry or fear about STDs to get in the way of the kind of sex life you want. Taking care of your sexual health need not be difficult or time-consuming, and sex between women remains the least 'risky' kind of sex anyone can have. Know about safer sex and be sensible about putting what you know into practice. Be familiar with your body and your partner's, and know how to get services if and when you need them. Play safe, stay well!

Further reading

Three essentials from Pat Califia

> *Sapphistry: The Book of Lesbian Sexuality* (Tallahassee: Naiad, 1988). Contains heaps of useful information, whatever your sexual preferences.

> *The Lesbian S/M Safety Manual* (Boston: Lace Publications/Alyson,1988). The essential safety guide for all dykes into S/M.

> *The Advocate Adviser* (Boston: Alyson,1991). Pat answers questions from readers of America's most widely read gay magazine.

Safer sex

> Cindy Patton and Janis Kelly, *Making It: A Woman's Guide to Sex in the Age of AIDS* (New York: Firebrand,1987). The first safe sex guide for women, and still one of the clearest.

> Diane Richardson, *Safer Sex: The Guide for Women Today* (London: Pandora,1990). Written by a lesbian, contains exhaustive information about HIV/AIDS and other safe sex issues for women having sex with women or men.

> Sue O'Sullivan and Pratibha Parmar, *Lesbians Talk (Safer) Sex* (London: Scarlet, 1992). Slender (and hence cheap!) discussion about HIV/AIDS and lesbians. Useful contacts and resources directory.

> If you cannot get your local feminist bookshop to touch Pat Califia with a barge pole (mine won't stock her books but, in the best tradition of pornographers everwhere, will order them for you and make you ask for them at the counter!), you can order them from: Gay's The Word, 66 Marchmont Street, London WC1N 1AB (tel.: 0171 278 7654).

4 A Tiny Bundle of Joy? Pregnancy, Birth and Parenting

The choice to have a child is never simple, and the processes of conception, birth and learning how to be a parent are complex and demanding for everyone, whatever their sexual identity. It is important that lesbians who travel this road do not fall into the trap of believing that every difficulty that arises can be put down to their sexuality. However, it is just as important for lesbians (and the professionals who provide services to us) to recognize that lesbian mothering brings its own set of problems and challenges. Most of these are minor and require only a little thoughtful advance planning to overcome, but some can be potentially devastating.

The market is flooded with books, videos and manuals which aim to help you become pregnant, have a 'good' pregnancy (however you define that), give birth in a positive way and bring up a happy, healthy child. With the exception of a pathetically tiny number, generally those written by feminists and/or lesbians, such books assume that mother or mother-to-be equals heterosexual and that parenting is something that takes place between a white, middle-class, severely able-bodied straight man and his white, middle-class, severely able-bodied straight female partner. They remain, nevertheless, useful sources of information. This chapter does not aim to replace the advice offered by these books (it does not, for example, discuss pain relief) but rather to offer some additional lesbian-specific material to help lesbians who want to negotiate their way through the maze of sometimes conflicting advice and to be prepared for some of the problems and joys of lesbian mothering.

Lesbian mothers:
mad, bad and dangerous to know?

There is *nothing* that distinguishes a lesbian pregnancy and birth from the non-lesbian equivalent. Nothing biological, that is; on the social and emotional level there is very little that is *not* different. Lesbian morning sickness is no different from heterosexual morning sickness and a lesbian contraction is indistinguishable from a heterosexual contraction. However, both are almost certainly *experienced* differently by lesbians, since the social and emotional meanings given to these physical events will be intimately affected by the social and emotional consequences of being a pregnant lesbian in a society which is deeply antagonistic to the very idea. The anxiety and exclusion felt by a lesbian non-biological co-parent is paralleled by the anxiety and exclusion felt by any new father, but springs from very different causes and will be felt in very different ways. For example, the biological father in a heterosexual couple has powerful legal rights over the child which the co-parent in a lesbian relationship does not, but a lesbian co-parent may be able to share breastfeeding of her child (see below), which a biological male cannot. We know very little about the impact of such complex issues on lesbian motherhood or co-parenting.

What we do know is that there is a great deal of hostility to the fact of lesbian motherhood. Throughout Britain, North America, Australasia and most of mainland Europe, lesbian mothers are faced with discriminatory laws, religious abhorrence, social intolerance and (especially in Britain) media outrage. Discrimination against lesbian mothers exists even in those supposedly liberal Scandinavian countries which have lesbian and gay partnership legislation. In Sweden, for example, lesbians and gay men may register their partnerships in a form of marriage but may not adopt children. What at first sight appears to be a tolerant acceptance of same-sex partnerships in fact has the consequence of officially identifying lesbians and gay men, thus making it much easier to prevent them adopting children.

There are plenty of causes for optimism. It is increasingly common in divorce proceedings for lesbian mothers to be awarded custody

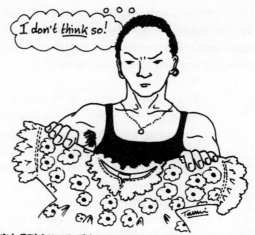

MARY SEARCHED THE CITY FOR A BUTCH LITTLE MATERNITY NUMBER.

of the children they gave birth to in heterosexual relationships; in some places (such as within some British local authorities) lesbians and gay men are considered suitable as adoptive and/or fostering candidates (although this all too often involves 'hard-to-place' children such as those with physical or intellectual impairments or with HIV). There is no doubt that the climate of opinion is shifting. Articles are starting to appear in the professional journals of midwives and nurse-midwives which aim to inform and educate about lesbian childbirth and parenting, and professional groups such as the Association of Radical Midwives are putting lesbian issues on their agenda. But the pace of change is frustratingly slow, especially for a woman who wants to have a baby before she retires!

The stigma against lesbian mothers is revealed when powerful individuals or groups take steps to prevent lesbians having children or keeping those they have. To understand it, we need to look closely at the stated reasons which have been given for denying lesbian mothers custody of their children, denying lesbians access to infertility treatment or denying lesbian co-parents access rights to their children when relationships break up. Unfortunately, there is a wealth of such material available, since judges, politicians and others are all too ready to articulate their distorted view on lesbians in public. Statements such as this are commonplace:

I don't say that a mother cannot be fit to rear her children even if she is a lesbian, but I wonder if she is fit when she boldly and brazenly sets up in the home where the children are to be reared, the lesbian practices which have been current there, clearly to the neglect of the supervision of the children.[1]

This judge's words give the key to the whole issue, namely that lesbianism is a *sexual* identity and that lesbians are assumed to be obsessed with the pursuit of perverted and secretive sexual pleasures. White Western culture has had enormous problems with reconciling the notion of motherhood with sexuality since before the Victorian era, and lesbian sexuality is particularly problematic. The very idea of female sexual behaviour which cannot lead to pregnancy, and hence cannot be explained away as a desire for babies rather than pleasure, challenges the centuries-old male myth that sexual pleasure is irrelevant to women and that pure, chaste motherhood is the height of female striving.[2] Most of the stated reasons for refusing to countenance lesbian motherhood spring from the definition of lesbianism as a sexual perversion. Such reasons have commonly included:

- the potential risk to the child's moral development of growing up in an 'immoral' environment

- the potential risk to the child of sexual abuse at the hands of its mother and/or any other sexual perverts that she happens to associate with

- the potential risk to the child of growing up lesbian or gay

- the potential risk to the child of growing up in a family situation which is seen as abnormal, and which may lead to the child being stigmatized or bullied at school

- the potential risk to the child of growing up without a father figure as a successful male role model

- the belief that lesbianism simply cannot co-exist with maternal feelings, since they are mutually contradictory and that therefore any lesbian will automatically be an 'unnatural' or unfit mother whether or not she has lesbian relationships.

We should not feel obliged to defend lesbian mothering against such slanders (especially since many of us would be delighted if our children grew up lesbian or gay!) but it is probably useful here to state unequivocally that a great deal of research has now been done on the children of lesbian mothers and *none* of the above accusations has any foundation whatsoever in real life.[3]

There are, however, two ways in which these outrageously silly beliefs may cause great damage to lesbian mothers and to our children. First, such beliefs continue to shape the decisions made by people who have the power to decide whether or not lesbians can have access to services such as donor insemination or fertility treatment, whether or not we can adopt or foster children and whether or not we are fit to be entrusted with the continuing care of those children we already have. Second, they place an enormous emotional burden on lesbians who want to be mothers, who are mothers or who are in parenting relationships with the children of partners or friends. These beliefs are widely current in the societies in which we live, and they affect us in two ways. First, it would be surprising if they didn't, at some level of our being, seriously undermine our own faith in our ability to care for children well. Second, we may well feel driven constantly to overcompensate, to be supermums whose every action is in the best interests of our children, in order to demonstrate to the world that lesbian mothering is beyond reproach. Mothering is difficult enough as it is, without having to shoulder extra burdens in this way! In addition, as many lesbian mothers will tell you, at the back of your mind is the constant awareness that your child may be taken away from you because you are a lesbian. Well-meaning non-lesbian friends don't really understand this one, and can often dismiss it as paranoia. But it isn't paranoia. However distant the possibility, every press report of another lesbian mother losing her child and every media frenzy against the spectre of lesbian motherhood reminds every lesbian mother that the risk is real.

These fears can have material consequences for the families of lesbians. Lesbians whose children come from previous heterosexual relationships or marriages may accept poor maintenance agreements and put up with lousy divorce settlements just to keep out of the courts.[4] Lesbian mothers who are entitled to state benefits may decide not to claim them, since they are fearful of drawing official attention to their status. Such factors must be seen in the context of other reasons why lesbian households are likely to be materially disadvantaged. First, there is the larger issue that women are more likely than men to be living in poverty, and that lesbians lack the access to a male wage that many (though not all) non-lesbian women take for granted. Second, lesbians are more likely than heterosexual women to be estranged from their families of origin, and this is likely to mean a reduction in the level of financial or material support available to bring up a child. It can be painful to witness the babies of heterosexual friends being showered with expensive gifts or even hand-me-downs from loving aunts, uncles and grandparents if your own family disowned you years ago on account of your sexuality.

Unity in oppression

So, those are some of the painful and difficult issues surrounding lesbian mothering. They will not all be true for all lesbians – for example, some of us are lucky enough to have loving and supportive parents – but any lesbian contemplating motherhood needs to be prepared to deal with the issues which she knows are likely to come up for her. It can be helpful to know that this degree of hostility is not reserved for lesbians. There are other groups of women who are often regarded as unfit mothers in white Western cultures, including disabled women, women of colour, women who use or are addicted to street drugs and women from the lower socio-economic groups. For example Susan Browne, Debra Connors and Nanci Stern write that:

Fear of disability and the belief that disability is inherited have led to judgements that disabled women should not be allowed to have children. We are actively discouraged from even considering the possibility. This is accomplished through the lack of appropriate sex education, forced sterilization, and the promotion of sterotypes that we are either asexual or sexually promiscuous.[5]

Sound familiar? Disabled women too may have to struggle to keep custody of their children[6] and may have to deal with the hostility of parents, family and society at large, including myths that it will be damaging to a child to be brought up by a disabled parent or parents.[7] The history of the forcible or coerced sterilization of First Nations' women, of women (and sometimes girl children) of colour and of women with intellectual impairments, and the widespread experimental use of injectable and implantable contraceptives on women in the 'Third' World should alert us to the fact that as lesbians we are not the *only* group which has to fight the idea that we should not be allowed to breed. It can be helpful understanding this, since it gives us a new perspective on all those destructive myths about lesbians being bad mothers. In whose interests is it that these myths are believed? The same people who spread the same myths about other oppressed groups of women. For black, minority or disabled lesbians, it can be tough disentangling the interwoven strands of the voices that repeat 'unfit mother', but it can also be exhilarating to recognize the same old attempts at social control (and racial purity) operating in a different guise. This recognition should be a powerful force for unity within the diverse lesbian community, and may offer a tool with which to challenge the homophobia of our other communities.

Moving away from the fraught social and emotional consequences of homophobia to the practicalities of lesbian mothering, what can be done to make the experience a good one for everyone involved? The rest of the chapter looks at conception, pregnancy, birth and becoming a parent.

Down to practicalities: getting ready to get pregnant

There is general agreement among midwives and others caring for birthing women and newborns that a woman who wishes to become a mother should start preparing her body several months *before* she gets pregnant. Increasingly, midwives and other professional childbirth specialists offer pre-pregnancy advice to women preparing for pregnancy; if this service is available to you, do take advantage of it.

This is the time when all the arguments about stress relief go out of the window and you *must give up smoking*. Every cigarette you smoke puts a strain on all the functions of your body, and if you smoke during pregnancy you will be forcing your growing baby to ingest powerful poisons at the time when its body is most vulnerable and sensitive, and when all its energies should be concentrated on the task of growth and development. Smoking is clearly linked to underweight babies, increased risk of stillbirth and of Sudden Infant Death Syndrome (cot death). You may be tempted by the myth it is easier to give birth to a small baby. Not true! The hard work and pain of labour is in the contractions which open the cervix, and the size of the baby makes no difference to that. If labour is managed well, there is no reason why birthing a full-sized baby should cause you to tear on delivery any more than an underweight baby. Indeed an underweight baby is more likely to be a weak baby and therefore more likely to need assistance at some time during the birth, either forceps delivery or artificial speeding-up of labour in order to get it delivered quickly if it is in distress. Bad news for the baby, bad news for you.

You should also give up any street drugs you are using – now is a good time to sign up for detox, since wanting a child can be a powerful motivation for successfully getting clean – and check with your doctor about the possible effects of any regular medication you are on for long-term health conditions. Some medications are potentially harmful, and may be replaced for the duration of your pregnancy by other, less harmful, alternatives. It may be useful to continue taking some – for example, if you have HIV and are taking AZT (Zidovudine), you may wish to discuss with your health care team the research which suggests that you may reduce the risks of transmitting HIV to your child if you continue to take AZT.

Alcohol is a less straightforward question. Native Americans will of course be aware of the problems associated with foetal alcohol syndrome, and the genetic predisposition of First Nations' people in America to alcoholism. But there is a degree of racism in the way this has been handled, and you should seek trusted advice when deciding whether or not to give up alcohol completely for the duration of your pregnancy.[8] Similarly, lesbians with a history of alcoholism in their family of origin or in themselves should seek trusted advice about this issue. For those whose drinking is usually light (a glass or two of wine, or a pint of beer or lager as a daily maximum) it is probably enough to make a slight reduction in this. Avoid spirits if possible, but do not feel that having an occasional glass of wine will damage your baby. However, drinking a lot *will* and, if you think you are drinking too much, get some help and support in dealing with it *before* you become pregnant.

You should also make every effort to eat as well as possible three or four months before trying to get pregnant, and during pregnancy. If you are seriously overweight, any weight that you are able to lose *before* becoming pregnant (do not attempt to lose weight once you are pregnant) will make pregnancy a much easier process for you. You should also take some exercise to try and strengthen your muscles and get fit, since pregnancy puts a strain on the body and the fitter you are, the easier it will be for you to cope with. Folic acid (a B vitamin) prevents anaemia and is essential to the healthy growth of the foetus; in Britain it is given in tablet form to all women from about the sixteenth week of pregnancy, but it is a good idea to increase your intake before pregnancy by incorporating it into your daily diet. Food sources of folic acid include green leafy vegetables such as cabbage or watercress (raw or lightly cooked), beans, lentils, peas, eggs, nuts, fruit and (fresh) fruit juices.

How to get pregnant

Getting pregnant is not biologically difficult. As Lisa Saffron says in her book on self-insemination, 'The procedure is so simple that it can be explained in one page, but the social and political consequences . . . fill this book.'[9] There are some fairly major choices to be made, which most non-lesbian women don't have to think about. If you are in a couple, the first question is which one of you is going to get pregnant. This is sometimes very straightforward; if one of you has always wanted to experience pregnancy and the other cannot think of anything worse (and this does not always divide neatly along butch/femme lines!) then you don't have a problem. For other women, the decision may be more complex, and the implications may feel daunting. The non-pregnant partner may anticipate having to deal with some painful jealousy – because her pregnant partner is getting all the attention, because of all the love, care and physical contact the baby will get from her partner, and because sex may take a back seat – and these are not the same in the context of a lesbian relationship as they are for men becoming fathers. On the other hand, the woman who becomes pregnant may feel very vulnerable and may fear abandonment or desertion by her non-pregnant partner. These are complex issues which need to be carefully talked through, with as much honesty as possible, *before* they become relationship emergencies.[10] Once you have decided who is going to become pregnant, you then have to decide *how* to go about making this happen. You have to decide on the method of semen delivery – are you going to have (unprotected, penetrative) sex with a man or are you going to use donated semen and inseminate without heterosex? Whichever you decide, there are then a whole host of other questions about the degree of involvement of the semen provider, all of which have legal and ethical implications. Taking all the variables into account, you have the following choices.

1. Having intercourse with a man who knows you are trying to get pregnant and who has agreed with you in advance that you will share parenting to a greater or lesser extent. *Questions to ask yourself: What happens if we disagree in future about our involvement in parenting? What if this man (or any current or future partner he may have) discovers unexpected feelings about the child once it is born? How will we both deal with the fact that he will have quite strong legal rights over the child? How will our involvement in parenting affect my current or any future lesbian relationships?*

2. Having intercourse with a man who knows you are trying to get pregnant and who has agreed with you in advance that he will have no further involvement in parenting. *Questions: All the above plus, what will happen if the child decides at some future date that it wants to meet its father?*

3. Having intercourse with a man who does not know you are trying to get pregnant and whom you do not intend telling if you do become pregnant. *Questions: How confident am I that I will be able to keep this knowledge from the man concerned? What will happen in the future if the child wants contact with its father? How will I go about getting the necessary health information about this man without letting him know what I intend? Am I happy that it is morally and ethically acceptable to do this, and what will happen if my feelings about this change once the child is born, or in future years?*

4. Using donated semen from a clinic or other formally registered establishment. *Questions: Will they provide services to lesbians? If not,*

how will I feel about pretending not to be a lesbian for the length of time it may take to get pregnant, and how will I do this? Can I afford the cost? (In the USA and Canada, donor insemination is rarely covered by health insurance, and the cost of getting pregnant can run into hundreds of dollars.)

5. Self-inseminating using semen from an anonymous donor and involving go-betweens in the collection of semen, health checks on donor(s), etc. *Questions: How will the go-between deal with the problem of knowing who I am and who the donor is, especially if the child wants in the future to contact its father? How will I feel if I accidentally discover the identity of the donor (especially if it is someone I dislike or I am related to)? How long will the donor and the go-between be prepared to go through the complex task of providing and delivering semen (it can take up to two years to get pregnant)?*

6. Self-insemination using semen from a known donor who will have no contact with the child in future. *Questions: as for (2).*

7. Self-insemination using semen from a known donor who agrees with you a negotiated sharing of childcare or other, more limited, contact with the child. *Questions: as for (1).*

8. Self-insemination with a fully co-parenting donor who will be fully involved in the care of the child. *Questions: As for (1), plus how is this going to affect my sense of myself as a lesbian, my relationship to the lesbian community and my current or future partner(s) and the nature of the parenting relationship in the eyes of the world? The world will treat the two of you as if you were a straightforward heterosexual couple, and the consequences of this are hard to predict!*

Once you have decided which to opt for, you need to consider the practicalities.

Getting pregnant through heterosex

If this is your first experience of having sex with a man, it makes sense to prepare yourself by talking to women friends who have had sex with men and/or by reading straight sex manuals. You need to decide how you will feel if the experience turns out to be sexually pleasurable or not. Will you try to enjoy it, or to be cold and clinical, and how can you prepare yourself emotionally for both these eventualities? You then need to check the health of the man involved (see below), and to check out with him that you both agree the limits of the experience. Remember that this may take several tries. Are you both prepared for the experience, and the possible consequences of having heterosex regularly for months?

Getting pregnant through donor insemination

If you are able to make use of the services of a clinic, much of the worrying will be done for you, and you can relax about many of the hassles such as legal issues, health checks, etc. But this can also lead you into taking a very passive role, and the whole experience may become uncomfortably clinical. Also, clinics which offer donor insemination are generally concerned with fertility 'treatment' and you may find that you are being treated as if you are infertile if you don't get pregnant pretty quickly.

If you are self-inseminating, you need to know as much as possible about the mechanics of conception. Conception takes place when an egg (or ovum) released from a woman's ovaries meets with a sperm from a man's semen (stored in the testicles/balls) and the sperm succeeds in entering the egg. From that moment the fertilized egg (a single cell) starts to divide, becomes implanted in the soft tissue lining the uterus/womb (it is this tissue which is shed every month during your period) and begins growing into a foetus. Of course you need to know when the egg is in the right place to be fertilized, and the semen needs to contain large numbers of live and healthy sperm. You will need to start charting your monthly fertile cycle for two or three months *before* you start inseminating. Generally your fertile period will be in the middle of your menstrual cycle, half-way between periods, but this is notoriously unreliable. There are physical signs that you have ovulated and are fertile. These include: the production of thin, clear, slippery fluid from your vagina, a rise in your basal body temperature, the neck of your womb (the cervix) lifting and moving further back in your vagina and (for some women) a sharp pain or mild, period-like cramps at the time of ovulation. You can now buy kits which tell you exactly when you are ovulating by using a simple urine test, but these are expensive and can make you very uptight and anxious. It is a good idea to get hold of some fairly detailed advice on how to recognize these signs and to become familiar with your own cycle.

To ensure that the semen is going to be useful it must be used before the sperm have become damaged or died. Ask your donor to ejaculate into a clean, wide-necked container such as a jam jar. Make sure that there are no traces of washing-up liquid or other cleaning materials in the container, since these may damage the sperm. Keep the semen at body temperature until it is to be used. If sperm become too hot, they will die (don't leave them in an airing cupboard or next to a stove or radiator). Try to use the semen within an hour, but bear in mind that sperm are quite robust and can probably cope with longer if need be.

You then need to get the semen as close to your cervix as possible, to give it a good change of swimming up and heading for the (hopefully) waiting egg. *Do not under any circumstances try to insert semen into your womb through the cervix*: it is not necessary and may be dangerous. It is perfectly adequate to place the semen high up in the vagina. You may self-inseminate using a meat baster (good for reaching high into the vagina, but tricky for getting the semen into), an eye-dropper (somewhat small, and putting glass into your vagina is probably not a good idea), a plastic cake-icing syringe (the range of nozzles can be helpful) or a plain medical syringe without a needle. A syringe is certainly the easiest thing to use, and getting hold of one is not as hard as it sounds. You can get one from most chemists/pharmacists. You won't necessarily want them to think you are injecting street drugs so try saying that you need it to give medicine to your guinea pig, to feed milk to an abandoned kitten, to fill your technical drawing pen with ink, etc. Or ask a friendly doctor, nurse or drugs project worker to get you one.

Lie on your back with your bottom propped up on a cushion, suck as much of the semen as possible up into your chosen instrument and insert it as far up into your vagina as you can reach. Tell yourself that this is a good time to get used to having strange objects inserted into your vagina. After all, you hope to be having a baby! It is a good idea to lie with your bottom on the cushion for as long as you can stave off boredom – twenty minutes minimum, half an hour should be plenty. If you have a partner who is involved, you may wish to combine the insemination with love-making. Indeed, if you are doing this alone you may still wish to make this an erotic or orgasmic moment. This is certainly not a necessity; if female sexual pleasure was necessary for conception the human species would have died out long ago! There is no firm evidence that having an orgasm helps fertilization, or that it makes you more likely to have a girl or a boy, but it can make the insemination feel more celebratory.

There are several things to remember about self-insemination. You should do it several times during each fertile period – three or four times if possible, and be prepared for it to take many months. It takes straight couples who are really trying hard an average of six months to conceive, and donor insemination generally takes longer. The chances of miscarriage or of a damaged foetus are no greater from donor insemination than from intercourse. Indeed, with your careful health checks, the risks may be slightly lower. But please also remember that miscarriage is *very* common – women tend to find out just how common when they become pregnant or have a miscarriage themselves. It is thought that up to a third of pregnancies miscarry spontaneously, many of them before the woman even realizes she is pregnant, so it is a good idea not to lose all contact with your donor and insemination support network the minute you get a positive pregnancy test.

How to tell when you are pregnant

Many women say they know they are pregnant before any test results. Certainly if you are trying to get pregnant, you will be focusing a lot of attention on your body. This may mean that you will know almost immediately, but it may also mean that every slight ache or sick feeling gets misinterpreted as a sign that you must be pregnant, and that can be miserably frustrating when your period starts as usual. Early signs can be heaviness, enlargement or soreness of your breasts, feelings of nausea (although these generally start later in the pregnancy) and a change in the scent of your urine, your sweat or your vaginal secretions.

If you think you are pregnant, you will probably want confirmation of this. Your local health centre will do a pregnancy test, as will any family planning clinic (in Britain) and some well woman clinics or centres offer this service too. You can, of course, buy your own pregnancy testing kits in a local chemist's shop or in many supermarkets, and this gives you the chance to confirm your suspicions yourself before telling anyone else. These kits are not expensive (although if you use one every month for several months to see if your insemination has worked, they can start to become expensive!); most are accurate as soon as two weeks after your first missed period.

If you are *not* pregnant, you may feel upset, confused, frustrated, cross or depressed. The longer you have been trying, the stronger such reactions may be. You may have to go through a process each time of grieving for *that particular baby*, the baby which didn't manage to get conceived this time. However rational and logical a person you are, the business of trying to have a child can kick off all sorts of seemingly irrational thoughts and emotions. The desire for a child can be as strong as any desire for a sexual partner, and you will need to take care of yourself during this time. If you are doing this on your own, make sure you have the support of at least one close and trusted friend who knows what you are doing. If you are doing it with a partner, both of you will have to pay attention to yourselves, each other and the relationship between you. Irritability, rows, irrational anger or grief may all be experienced at this time.

If you are pregnant, you may want to wait a few weeks or months before telling people the glad tidings. The possibility of miscarriage is at its highest in the first three months, and, whilst you will of course want to tell those closest to you, it may be worth waiting until the pregnancy is well established before breaking the news to others less closely involved.

What to do during pregnancy

This is the point to go out and get a good pregnancy book, one that is recommended by friends, and to start taking care of yourself. Pregnancy is divided up by health professionals into three *trimesters* (three-month blocks). Most of the hard work that your body has to do adjusting to being pregnant takes place in the first trimester. This can feel grossly unfair. Your hormones have gone crazy, you may be feeling exhausted, tearful, nauseous and scared and there is not so much as a bump in your tummy to alert others to your need to be taken care of! Many women sail through with no problems at all, but others may experience a miserable depression (a little like being pre-menstrual for three months), and some women have really horrible morning sickness. Ignore anyone who tries to tell you that morning sickness is all in your mind and is caused by you fighting the idea of becoming a mother. There are studies showing that women in some cultures don't experience morning sickness, but that doesn't prove that it is psychosomatic! If you get morning sickness badly (and some women get it throughout the day, not just on waking), try to note whether anything makes it worse. Some foods or drinks may become hard to tolerate, and others may be very helpful. My own experience was that the recommended solution (a cup of tea and a dry biscuit first thing in the morning) made me throw up faster than anything, but other women swear by it. Morning sickness usually wears off after the first trimester, but for a few very unlucky women it can last for their entire pregnancy. If this happens to you, don't let anyone tell you that it means that you don't want the baby or that, as a lesbian, it is unnatural or difficult for you to do such a normal, female thing as being pregnant. It just means that this is the way your body happens to respond to the stresses and changes of pregnancy, and you are simply unlucky. Unless you are one of those rare and unfortunate women whose sickness is *very* severe (severe enough to cause you to lose large amounts of weight) you should avoid taking anti-nausea drugs.

Lesbian sex in pregnancy

When you become pregnant, you will discover that pregnancy affects almost every part of your body, and some you didn't know you had. Did you know, for example, that the veins on your forearms enlarge in order to dissipate the extra heat caused by the foetus? Or that the shape of your eyeballs changes as the fluid inside them increases? It also has unpredictable effects on your emotional life and on your sexuality. Some women go right off sex for some or all of the time, others become ravenously sexual. As you get larger, and especially in the third trimester, your feet and legs may ache and swell from the extra weight, your pelvis begins to change shape as the joints loosen to get ready for birth, and you may get strange pains in your belly, your vagina or your breasts. You will almost certainly experience uterine contractions as the time for birth approaches. These are called 'Braxton-Hicks contractions' and are nothing to worry about. Some women find that orgasm (which can make your whole 'bump' go rigid in a quite alarming way) sets these contractions off. But orgasm will not cause you to go into labour unless you were about to anyway, so there is no need to give up sex.

Although most pregnancy and childbirth handbooks are reassuring about continuing sexual activity throughout pregnancy, I have yet to find one which mentions lesbian sex in this context. However, it is possible to look at the advice given in these books and draw reasonably accurate conclusions about lesbian sexual activities. During pregnancy the growing foetus is very securely held in its sac of amniotic fluid inside the uterus and is unlikely to be dislodged by sexual activity on the part of the mother. The exception to this is where the cervix has been damaged (perhaps during a mismanaged abortion) or is (in dreadful medical language) 'incompetent'. If your cervix is 'incompetent' you are most likely to find this out from repeated miscarriages. Women with this kind of cervical weakness may have a 'purse-string' stitch inserted to hold the cervix closed as the foetus becomes larger, and may have to spend the large part of their pregnancy resting or lying in bed. Under these stressful circumstances you are unlikely to want to take the risk of lovemaking, and will certainly want detailed and explicit advice from your doctor or midwife if you do decide to go ahead.

During a more routine pregnancy, however, most lesbian sexual activities are highly unlikely to cause problems. There is no need to worry about orgasms, oral sex, any form of clitoral stimulation or inserting fingers, tongues, etc. into the vagina. If you are into penetration with something bigger, a dildo for example, it is a good idea to be particularly careful to avoid infection. Wash your sex toys regularly, don't share them between users without either washing them in between or using a fresh condom, and *never* put anything in a vagina which has been in an anus without thorough washing. You may find that you want a smaller dildo than usual, and certainly you should not use one which is large enough to cause pain. You may prefer not to bump your cervix while you are pregnant, but don't worry if you do. Using butt plugs or using a dildo in the anus may be uncomfortable during the later stages. Be aware that all your internal organs get squashed and shifted out of place as the foetus grows, and that you may bruise something which is usually out of reach; it makes sense to be more cautious than usual with dildos and butt plugs, but it is safe to let your own comfort be your guide. If you enjoy vaginal fisting, it is probably best avoided as the foetus grows, simply because you are likely to feel bruised and sore anyway, and it is less easy to tell if you are causing additional bruising. Anal fisting should be *avoided* during pregnancy, since the risk of damage and peritonitis is simply not worth taking at this time.

You may find your breasts and nipples are extra-sensitive, or they may be too painful to touch. As pregnancy advances, your breasts may start to produce milk, and this can leak out if your nipples are sucked or played with. Whether this is a problem or not is entirely up to you and your lover – it won't do any harm. Because the number of nerve endings in your belly does not increase as it expands, having someone stroke your belly while you shut your eyes can be a strange experience, since your brain tells you it is the familar, pre-pregnancy shape and size. This expanding belly will be the thing you have to deal with during sex. Straight childbirth manuals often illustrate different positions for sex for a pregnant woman. Because of the more varied options open for lesbian sex, this tends to be less of a problem for lesbian lovers, but you still need to be careful not to put weight on the 'bump', and a pregnant woman may find it too uncomfortable to lie on her stomach once the pregnancy starts to show. *If you are into sadomasochism, you should never whip, burn, cut or beat a pregnant woman's belly, vulva or breasts, and she should not be tied up for more than a few minutes. Nor should you do piercings at this time.* Sadomasochistic sex play should be reduced to a near-vanilla level during pregnancy. Rituals involving humiliation or servility may also take on a very different emotional tone for a pregnant woman, and you should take greater care than usual to stay alert for signs that this is not play any more. However, pregnancy gives some women immense feelings of power and strength, and there is no reason why a pregnant woman should not make a great top!

Childbirth classes

Going to childbirth classes can be very useful but it is all too often a depressingly heterosexist environment. Childbirth or parentcraft sessions run by health care professionals are often free and will give you useful basic information, or there may be some classes run by voluntary groups in your area. In Britain the National Childbirth Trust (NCT) runs classes which give very detailed information and support and teach breathing exercises for pain control. There is a charge for these, they become booked up very fast and they are usually very middle-class, but you will meet a group of other mothers who may become an invaluable support and friendship network during pregnancy and early motherhood. This can be important, since most lesbian communities are ill-equipped to support new mothers. My son is fifteen years old, and I am still in contact with women I met during NCT childbirth classes. It is also important to find out during your pregnancy what support is available for breastfeeding. Hospital staff and even many midwives are extraordinarily ill-informed about successful breastfeeding, and it is very useful to have contact with someone who knows how to help you get started. A friend who has successfully breastfed may be more useful than all the obstetric nurses in the world.

Birth

There is nothing that quite compares with the knowledge that you are going to give birth. If you have not done it before, you have the anxiety of knowing that you are inevitably drawing closer to an unknown experience that will include a kind of pain you are unfamiliar with, that you don't have any idea whether you can cope with and that will end up by moving your baby out of the safety of your womb into the world where s/he will need your attentive care – changing your life for ever. One factor that can make all the difference in your experience of birth is the place of birth. Home birth is preferred by many women and offers important additional advantages for lesbians. You will be less likely to have to deal with homophobic staff, you will have more control over who is present and, unless there is good reason to foresee complications, it is perfectly safe. To find out whether this is an option for you, check with local midwives and with your doctor. You may also want to consider possibilities such as the use of birthing stools, a water birth or using a birthing centre. The availability of such options varies greatly from place to place, and should be talked through with as many people as possible. If you decide to opt for a hospital delivery, you should carefully discuss who you want to be present. You do not, for example, have to agree to allow students to observe if you do not want to.

Nobody can prepare you for the sensations of birth. For some women it is an extremely strong physical task that bears no relationship to anything they would call 'pain'; for others it is very painful indeed. Some women sail through in eight or nine hours, happily doing their breathing exercises, while others are lumbered with twenty hours or more. Some find back rubs and warm flannels enough, others opt for spinal block anaesthetic or end up having caesarians. You can't predict what your experience will be. But it does help to know what is happening, and to try to work with that rather than panic and work against it.

What happens

Labour is divided into stages, and each stage requires something different from you. The first stage is generally the longest, and involves the cervix being opened wide enough to allow the baby to be pushed out into the world. If you remember that the cervical os, a tiny hole that is normally smaller than the tip of a biro, is being slowly and gradually stretched to the size where it can allow the baby's head through, you will be able to make sense of the physical sensations. The contractions that draw back and open the cervix are extraordinarily strong, and there is no doubt that most women experience them as painful. However, by concentrating on visualizing what each contraction is doing, and by relaxing and letting your body get on with it, you may well find you need no pain relief at all. If you hate the sensations and find yourself resisting them, or if you are the kind of person who hates feeling out of control, you may want to opt for pain relief at this point.

The pain can feel worse if the baby is in an unusual position, if it is breech (bottom-first) or posterior (with the wide part of its head presenting) for example. If this is the case, try experimenting with different positions. Lie on your side, crouch, go on all fours, kneel or walk around. You may find that a simple change of position is all that is needed to make things much easier. If you have the opportunity to use a birthing pool (available in many birthing centres and in some enlightened maternity hospitals), getting into the water can be enough to make the contractions immediately less painful and more easy to work with.

The next stage is when the baby moves out of the uterus and into the vagina, ready to be pushed out. There may be a 'transition' stage between the two, which may cause you to become very shaky, chilled, panicky, tearful or irritable. Transition is recognized to be a difficult moment in labour, and a competent birthing helper should recognize it and remind you what is happening. It is in fact a good sign, since it tells you that the long, hard slog of the first stage is over, and the baby will soon be with you! You may feel an urge to push during transition. This is misnamed, since it can feel almost as if your body has taken over completely and has decided to push anyway, with or without your will. It can be very hard to stop yourself from pushing at this point, but you should pay attention to the advice of your birthing helper, since pushing too soon (perhaps before the baby is fully into the vagina) is unhelpful.

Many women, especially women who are unfit, chronically ill or have some physical impairment, wonder whether they will have the strength to push the baby out. The answer is that you don't have to. Just keep relaxing and letting your body do all the work. It helps to be as upright as possible during this stage, so you should resist any attempts to get you on your back with your feet in stirrups, unless there is very good reason (for example, forceps delivery during an obstructed labour or to get a distressed baby out fast). If you have chosen an epidural, you may find that it does not wear off fast enough for you to deliver the baby successfully. Don't panic, the baby will get born!

At some point, probably when you have forgotten what this is all about anyway, your birthing attendants will tell you excitedly that they can see the baby's head (or bottom if it is breech). Put your hand down and touch it, or ask for a mirror so that you can see it too. There is no excitement to compare with that first contact between you and this baby who has been a mystery for so long, and there is nothing like being able to touch the head to dispel the exhaustion of labour and speed you through the delivery.

You should be able to deliver the baby with little or no tearing to your vagina. If the baby is very large or if forceps become necessary, you may have an episiotomy, a cut made in the perineum below and to one side of the vagina. This is a drag, since it needs stitching after the birth and will be sore for several days until it heals and the stitches can be removed, but if it is skilfully mended afterwards it need not be a problem. Some birthing positions can greatly reduce the risk of tearing: sitting propped up in bed gives the least amount of room for the baby, and it is much better to stand up, squat, get on to all fours or lie on your left side. Your birthing attendant should be able to help at this point.

Once the baby is in your arms, you will find that s/he may be covered with a pale grease called *vernix*, which protects the skin from the amniotic fluid, that s/he may be an odd colour or that s/he may be a little squashed-looking from the birth. Put to your nipple, the baby should start to suck straight away. At some point you will then go into the next stage, when the placenta, looking like an enormous piece of liver, is delivered. This is the organ which has developed during the pregnancy to nourish the baby, and it generally turns up just after the baby, with its own contractions. Some birthing assistants pull it out with a process called 'controlled cord traction' (CCT), which requires an injection to aid the process. CCT is usually unnecessary and may result in bleeding or in pieces of the placenta being left behind, but it can speed things up. You should make it clear before you go into labour if you do not want it done (unless for some reason it becomes necessary). Once the placenta is delivered, it will be thoroughly checked to make sure that it is in one piece, since any fragments left in the uterus may cause infection later on.

If you have torn during the birth, or if you have been given an episiotomy, you will be stitched at this point. If you have had an epidural, you may not need any additional anaesthetic for the stitching, but do not be shy about asking to be given one anyway if you are concerned. The skills of the person doing the stitching will have important consequences for how quickly you heal, how much pain you experience during the first few days following the birth, and on any scarring later (which can have an impact on your sex life – sometimes a tight episiotomy or a bad scar can make penetration painful), so it is reasonable to ask not to be stitched by a student.[11]

The end and the beginning: being a new lesbian mother

It is not surprising that, during pregnancy, birth is seen as the outcome of the whole process. Once you have produced a baby, the realization that this is the beginning of a lifetime's relationship gradually dawns. It can hit some women at once, as this lesbian mother relates:

> 66 Once he was born I was exhausted and didn't really care whether I'd given birth to a baby or a garden shed, but when he was put into my arms and our eyes met for the first time I was shocked to the core of my being by the realization that he looked like me. It sounds so silly, but in that instant I fully grasped for the first time the significance of what I had done. This child was connected to me, to who I am, and to my body, in a way that I hadn't anticipated. Even now, when he's taller than me, it hits me sometimes. You can't explain it, you really can't. 99

> 'Dawn'

For some, the dawning realization of just how responsible a mother is for her newborn is exciting, exhilarating and warming; for others it can be sickeningly frightening, especially if we are giving birth outside a secure love relationship or in a relationship that we know or fear to be fragile. Since lesbian relationships lack the powerful legal, cultural and social support given to heterosexual relationships or marriages, and since we are not supposed to be able to look after children anyway, this time can be especially scary for lesbian mothers, whether or not they have lovers and/or co-parents. All sorts of painful questions, doubts and fantasies may come up, either soon after the birth or during the weeks and months to come. It probably doesn't help to dismiss these fears; however irrational they may seem, they are often clues to very real and well-founded anxieties. It helps to know that they almost certainly *will* surface, and to have access to sympathetic friends who will listen without feeling that they have to calm you down or solve your problems. If you have worked with a counsellor or therapist in the past and found this helpful, by all means make use of this coping strategy; this can be especially useful if you are offloading everything on to your partner, since she will be needing as much support as she can get in adjusting to her changing status as well.

Practicalities: food and sleep

Once the baby is born, it can seem as if all the love and attention which you received when you were pregnant is now suddenly taken away from you and given to the baby. Caring for your own needs, and asking others to recognize those needs, is especially important at this time. Food and sleep for you and the baby usually take over the first few months. It is unlikely that you will be able to do anything about this, and it is better to give in than to expend precious energy fighting it!

I have to admit at this point that I am a breastfeeding fanatic. If they ever bring back wet nursing, I shall be first in the queue. I found breastfeeding a complete delight. It didn't turn me on or give me orgasms (a prospect that had alarmed me somewhat during pregnancy!) but it gave me a delightful sensual pleasure and a great sense of achievement. To hear your baby swallowing noisily and know that you are producing enough milk to keep her or him gulping away is a great thrill. But the most wonderful thing is that it is so practical. It is far and away the best food for your baby, being custom-made for the purpose and chock-full of all the complex antibodies, vitamins and proteins s/he needs to develop a fully functioning immune system and to grow in the right way. It is also no bother to prepare or provide. If your baby sleeps in with you, night feeds may hardly disturb your sleep, since you just need to roll over and let the baby suck on demand. When you are out together, you can breastfeed almost unnoticed if you carry the baby in a sling and simply undo a shirt button or roll up your sweatshirt when s/he is hungry. If you use a sling in this way, you can carry on doing almost anything while feeding your baby. I have hoovered, done the supermarket shopping, washed the dishes, helped extract honey from beehives and painted shelves while breastfeeding.

All of which sounds positively idyllic, but of course things don't feel like that to start with. The force with which a newborn sucks on the nipple can be startling, and it may be painful unless s/he has enough of your nipple in the mouth. It is not enough to suck on the tip, the baby needs to get a full mouthful of the breast. You will probably get sore nipples anyway for the first few days, although this soreness generally needs no treatment. You can prevent cracked nipples by getting the baby properly 'latched on', by not washing your nipples too much (you don't need to wash them at all, other than as you usually would in your regular bath/shower), by applying a gentle ointment such as calendula or cocoa butter between feeds for the first few days and by removing the baby from your breast *gently*. Break the suction by gently inserting the tip of your little finger in the corner of his/her mouth if you want her/him to stop sucking.

Another problem is that the closeness of breastfeeding can be very excluding for lovers and co-parents. This is where lesbian mothering offers a great advantage over heterosexual parenting, since a non-biological co-mother can, if she wishes, eventually produce milk and share in the breastfeeding of her baby. There is a device called the 'Lact-Aid', which is basically a milk reservoir attached to a thin tube. You fix the tube to your nipple and fill the reservoir with expressed breast milk. The sucking baby then gets fed, and the continual sucking will eventually stimulate your breasts to produce milk. This takes time; if you are interested, you will need the support of a counsellor from the La Leche League (which exists to promote breastfeeding) or a breastfeeding counsellor from the NCT or your birthing centre. Even if the co-mother does not want to lactate, allowing the baby to suck her nipples will often stop him/her crying and comfort the baby if it is unhappy or sleepy (although not, of course, if s/he is hungry, in which case s/he will suck for a while and then howl in outrage!).

If you breastfeed, you may find that your baby is allergic to cow's milk. This allergy produces what is sometimes called 'three-month colic'. Some health care professionals believe that all babies get three-month colic, during which they scream and cry and are unpacifiable for days or weeks. Women in Scandinavian countries cannot understand why this is allowed to happen, since they believe that this fretful crying is a reaction to cow's milk. If it happens to your baby, try cutting cow's milk and dairy products out of your diet altogether. The results can be miraculous. You can then 'test' the baby at monthly intervals, by having a milky drink and observing the baby's reaction. If this doesn't solve the problem, or if you feel that there is something seriously wrong with your baby, don't hesitate to seek medical advice.

If you don't want to breastfeed, then formula feeding is a safe option in industrialized nations (although not in poor nations of the 'Third World', where bottlefeeding causes many thousands of infant deaths every year). You will need sterilizing equipment, at least six bottles and teats the right size for your baby's age, and a supply of formula and clean water. Some women prefer to filter water to be used in baby feeding, since it removes some of the harmful trace elements in tap water, but you should *not* use bottled or mineral water. You should always read and follow instructions for sterilizing equipment, and for preparing feeds. *Never* use either more or less formula than the manufacturer instructs on the packet, since these proportions are carefully developed to produce feeds of the right strength for infants at different ages. If you decide to bottlefeed, you should try to breastfeed for at least the first week if at all possible, since it is at this time that your baby will get the 'colostrum' – an extra-rich food intended for newborns – and will get at least some of the antibodies and proteins which s/he needs in those vulnerable early days.

Bottlefeeding has the undoubted advantage that anyone can do it, so you are able to share care of your baby around much more widely than you would otherwise. Only you can weigh up the pros and cons of breast and bottle. However, it is much easier to change your mind from breastfeeding to bottlefeeding than the other way round. If you start off bottlefeeding and then decide that you would rather give breastfeeding a go, you may find it very difficult to establish your milk supply (depending on how long you have gone without breastfeeding), and to teach the baby a very different way of sucking. Whatever decision you make, it helps enormously to have the support of someone who has successfully breastfed, since you are then able to be much clearer about what you are basing your choice on.

Feeding yourself

You may not have much appetite for a few days after the birth, owing to the physical and emotional adjustments you are making, or you may eat like a horse! Whichever applies to you, you need at this time to eat as well as you can afford to, and to be looked after as much as possible by others. Now is the time to take people up on their offers of help. Ask friends and relatives to cook a meal for you, or to bring food with them when they visit the new baby. You should eat plenty of fresh fruit and vegetables, as much protein as possible, and plenty of complex carbohydrate, as well as foods which are rich in iron and other minerals. If you are breastfeeding, you will find that your nutrition needs are greater than usual, and you will probably feel thirstier. Drink more fresh water, fruit juice and (unless your baby is allergic to it) milk. Do not worry about 'losing the weight you put on during pregnancy' while you have to have the energy to care for a newborn or a demanding infant, and *do not try to lose weight while breastfeeding*, although many women find that they do anyway.

Sleep

Stopping people sleeping is a form of torture used with great success by repressive regimes, a fact that you will understand only too well after the first few weeks with a newborn. Babies are not born attuned to the rhythm of day and night. They are born attuned to the demands of a tiny stomach, which can hold only enough food to keep them going for a few hours. What is more, they don't understand what hunger is, and they have no means of knowing that you are around to make sure they don't die of starvation. Feeling empty is terrifying for a tiny baby, and when the baby is hungry s/he will cry, urgently. For the first few weeks, this means that for you, too, day and night will lose their familiar shape, and you will become tired and disorientated. Some lucky women take this in their stride, but you may be horrified at how sleep deprivation makes you feel. You've just been through nine months of pregnancy and an exhausting labour, can't the child leave you in peace for just one night? You may feel resentful, angry and despairing, or as if you want to give the baby away and forget you ever had her or him. You may desperately yearn for some uninterrupted high-quality time with your partner, and wonder if you will ever get it again.

There are many ways of making this time easier. Sleeping with the baby makes it easy to give him/her the breast without even waking up properly – although until you have got used to breastfeeding it won't be quite as easy as that; if you are bottlefeeding, refrigerating enough made-up formula feeds for the night before you go to bed will reduce the amount of time you have to spend trying to pacify a hungry baby while you rinse out bottles from the sterilizer. Above all, accept that it is going to be like this for a while, and plan your life around it. This bit lasts only a few weeks, so put off returning to work, sleep as much as you can during the day, get friends and family in to do the housework so you can rest, and try to see this as a special and precious chunk of 'time out' from the rest of your life.

More issues for lesbians: taking steps to make life easier

It may seem as though this process of adjustment after your baby is born is little different from the process that non-lesbian mothers have to go through. In many ways this is true, but it is important that lesbian mothers, their friends and communities and the health professionals who provide services to lesbian clients should all recognize that this process contains additional stresses for lesbians. There is not the same unambiguous support on offer to lesbian mothers as there is available to most non-lesbian women. First, the pressure that homophobia and the widespread hostility to lesbian mothering exerts on lesbian mothers, their co-parents and partners and (at a later time) their children should not be underestimated. Feelings of doubt in our ability to mother, of guilt that the child has had no choice about being brought into the world under such problematic circumstances, or of fear that we may lose custody are among the additional difficulties that homophobia introduces into lesbian mothers' lives. Second, support from other lesbians may not be forthcoming. A larger proportion of lesbians are childless, and the business of birth and childrearing sits less easily with the daily preoccupations of many lesbian communities. A minority of revolutionary separatist lesbian feminists are extremely hostile to lesbians having children,[12] and the relative rarity of lesbian mothers means that many of our support networks inevitably include non-lesbian women, who are, however well-meaning, unlikely to have any realistic understanding of what being a lesbian mother involves. It is important to establish as wide a network of support as possible, as early in the pregnancy as possible, so that some of these difficulties may be overcome. Setting up baby-sitting circles with other mothers may mean, for example, deciding how you feel about non-lesbian women's male partners being involved in the care of your child. Many men provide excellent care for infants, but only you can decide on whether or not you are happy with this, and it is best to decide *before* the situation arises, rather than risk hurting or offending your straight friends.

Sex after birth

Most childbirth books include information about resuming heterosexual activity after birth, but I have not been able to track down any information about lesbian sex! It is safest to let your body and your desires be your guide. Of course, penetration will be out of the question for a while, but there is no hard and fast rule about when it becomes OK, so take it gently and let your body guide you. If you have had a lot of stitches or much bruising, you may feel pretty traumatized and vulnerable, and even the easiest of births will leave you with a legacy of exhaustion and depletion. You may have very new feelings about your body, which can seem strange and alien as it makes rapid transitions from being hugely pregnant to being squidgy and sore, to gradually recovering a more familiar shape. You may feel sad or elated about your stretch marks and your big, milky, large-veined breasts with their tendency to leak at odd moments. But if you pay caring attention to how you are feeling, both physically and emotionally, then you should have the kind of sex that you want, when you feel ready. Don't be surprised if you are in need of frequent hugs and cuddles, or if, on the other hand, you are less willing to be touched. You will recover from the physical and emotional experience of birth in your own way. Faced with a lover who is desperate for sex and finding it hard to take a slow pace, you may like to use some of the strategies recommended for ill or disabled women in Chapter 7.

Getting good care

Simply ensuring good health care services during pregnancy and birth or for your growing infant is more difficult for lesbians. Research shows that lesbians are more likely to receive poor care:

Because of the paucity of information about the dilemmas and needs of childbearing lesbians, along with blatant discrimination and prejudiced attitudes, lesbian childbearing couples are at risk for receiving less than optimal health care.[13]

This can include insulting or nervous behaviour from nurses, midwives, health visitors or doctors so subtle as to leave you unsure whether or not you are imagining it, but it can be extreme. In one study carried out in the USA in 1989, eleven per cent of lesbians interviewed were actually *refused antenatal care* by health care practitioners.[14] In Britain the practice of health visitors making regular visits to check on the progress of the infant, and to support the mother adjusting to her new role, can be a welcome source of support. For some mothers, however, it can feel uncomfortably like surveillance, and can certainly feel as if someone is judging your competence to be a mother. For women in some minority ethnic communities, or women who are poor or otherwise disadvantaged, this can be very undermining. For some groups of women, in particular mothers with moderate to severe physical or intellectual impairments, it can seem like a routine trial. For lesbians, contact with a possibly homophobic health visitor may be extremely frightening, since there is always the fear that the state may intervene to remove your child. This fear is largely unfounded, since health visitors do not have that kind of legal power, but a hostile one can be very undermining. However, most health vistors are doing the job because they have a genuine concern for the health and wellbeing of infants and mothers, and if you establish a friendly relationship with yours, she may be a useful ally, able to offer much-needed support and to inform you about services and benefits to which you may be entitled. Outside Britain, where there is no health visitor service, you may be able to get this kind of advice from a women's health centre, midwife or local support group.

The future

Becoming a mother has lifelong implications for all women, but those implications are very different for lesbians. Your baby will change your life irrevocably. S/he will change your idea of yourself as a lesbian, your relationship with your lesbian friends, partner(s) and community, your family, your workmates and even your pets. You will be confronted at times with the realities of homophobia, and there are times when this causes very real material difficulties. As two researchers remind us, this can be especially true in countries that lack properly funded state health care:

Many biological lesbian mothers feel impelled to work to obtain health care insurance for themselves and their children. Because lesbian partners cannot be on each others' health insurance policies, and the nonbiological parent cannot have the child on her health plan, the biological parent cannot afford to be unemployed if she wants her child to receive the benefits and protections health insurance offers.[15]

In addition, you will have to confront the homophobia your child faces as the child of a lesbian mother, and will have to find a way to make her or him feel OK in the face of a cultural onslaught of images and words which tell her or him constantly that a 'proper' family has a mum, a dad and 2.4 children. But you will also know that having you as a mother offers many special advantages. Your child will be less likely to be sexually abused, since 'the evidence is that children, especially girls, being brought up in a lesbian household are at far less risk of sexual abuse than children raised in a household with a male parent present.[16] What is more, children raised in lesbian households are likely to have a head start when it comes to establishing relationships with a diverse range of people. They will be practised in questioning the received wisdom of the mainstream, may be more sophisticated in their understandings of stereotyping, stigma and scapegoating, and may be able to see themselves as 'special' rather than 'weird'. They will almost certainly give you a hard time about your sexuality at some point in their lives, but don't forget that *all* children do that to a greater or lesser extent. As lesbian mothers we may have something very precious to offer our children, and there are certainly enormous pleasures which they bring to us.

Further reading

The best guide for lesbians trying to get pregnant is Lisa Saffron's book *Challenging Conceptions: Planning a Family by Self-Insemination* (London: Cassell,1994).

For detailed discussion about pregnancy, labour, birth, pain relief and other issues, go for Boston Women's Health Book Collective (eds), *The New Our Bodies Ourselves* (Harmondsworth: Penguin,1989).

For advice and information on becoming a mother later in life, see Jean Shapiro, *Ourselves, Growing Older: Women Ageing with Knowledge and Power* (London: Fontana,1988).

Books on the business of lesbian parenting, and on what it is like to be the child of a lesbian parent include:

Katherine Arnup, *Lesbian Parenting: Living with Pride and Prejudice* (San Francisco: Gynergy Books, 1995).

Sandra Pollack and Jeanne Vaughan (eds), *Politics of the Heart: A Lesbian Parenting Anthology* (New York: Firebrand,1987).

April Martin, *The Guide to Lesbian and Gay Parenting* (London: Pandora,1993).

Harriet Alpert, *We Are Everywhere: Writings by and about Lesbian Parents* (Boston: The Crossing Press, 1988).

Louise Rafkin, *Different Mothers: Sons and Daughters of Lesbians Talk About their Lives* (San Francisco: Cleis Press, 1989).

5 Out of Mind, Out of Sight? Mental and Emotional Health

The field of mental health is fraught with difficulties for lesbians. Many of these difficulties spring from the high level of stigma which is still attached to those who experience periods of 'mental illness'. It seems ironic that this stigma should remain so intense when statistics show that mental illness (or, at least, what medical science calls mental illness) is extremely common. In Britain, for example, surveys typically report that 'about 70% of women and 50% of men will at some time in their lives consult their general practitioner about a mental health problem',[1] while as many as one in nine men and one in six women will spend some time in a psychiatric institution.[2] When an experience is so widespread that it affects more than half the population it begins to seem normal rather than abnormal. Yet the intensity of the stigma attached to mental illness is self-perpetuating. Many people who have recovered from an experience which was diagnosed as a mental illness not only wish to move on swiftly from an intrinsically unpleasant time in their lives but also soon recognize that 'coming out' as an ex-psychiatric patient is so stigmatizing that it is in their best interests to keep the knowledge as secret as possible.

In this sense, being a 'mental patient' has much in common with being a lesbian, and some of the consequences are similar. Like lesbianism, mental illness is a stigmatizing label, and so, like lesbians, individuals who have been labelled mentally ill tend to remain hidden and to hide this part of their identity. The political activism of mental health advocacy groups includes the strategy of speaking out by survivors of the psychiatric system, which has clear parallels with the gay liberationist strategy of coming out. Mental health system survivors, however, remain one of the most disenfranchised of political activist groups, and this has important consequences for lesbians who experience emotional or mental distress or disturbance, since there continues to be a profound silence surrounding the mental health needs and experiences of lesbians.

As usual, this silence is twofold. There is now an extensive body of feminist work on women's mental health and a growing body of 'gay-affirmative' work on lesbian and gay mental health. Surprise, surprise, the feminist work tends to concentrate on heterosexual women and the gay work tends to concentrate on men. Lesbians fall down that oh, so familar hole in the middle. This chapter therefore has two jobs to do: first to explain some of the key issues in lesbian mental health and second to offer some practical suggestions for lesbians struggling with mental health problems. The second task is more important to users of this book but it makes no sense without an understanding of the wider issues, so I will start with a discussion of these.

Key issues in lesbian mental health

It is important to understand that the very idea of mental illness is one which we cannot take for granted. It is based on the idea that there is something called variously the mind, the personality or the identity, which can become diseased or start to go wrong. This is not an idea that is accepted by everyone, although it guides the practice of mental health professionals in the medical industry and many counsellors, psychotherapists or alternative healers. An alternative proposition is that what doctors and psychiatrists label 'symptoms' of mental 'illness' are in fact quite rational responses, or even coping strategies, which people adopt when faced with intolerable or damaging situations. Those who hold such beliefs tend to refer to mental or emotional 'distress' rather than illness. It is probably fair to say that there is an element of truth in both positions. Madness is not a well-funded area of medical research or health care; it tends to be seen as low-priority (partly because it is so difficult to 'cure') and one result is that we have a very limited understanding of this field of human suffering. There do, however, appear to be some conditions which make sense when you try to understand them as an illness. Some of the serious, long-lasting conditions generally called *psychoses* fall into this category. These include conditions such as schizophrenia, and people suffering from them often get great relief from medical treatment, including some of the newer drugs. However, even 'serious' mental illness is often very clearly linked to social factors in ways which cannot be explained by the idea that it is an illness. For example, Afro-Caribbean men in Britain are enormously over-represented in diagnoses of schizophrenia, and critics have pointed out that this is likely to have much to do with racist attitudes, the misinterpretation of culturally specific expressions of distress, and (not least) the routine harassment of black men by the police. Activists in the anti-psychiatry movement in the 1960s and 1970s, who include such writers as Thomas Szasz and R. D. Laing, insisted that even the 'symptoms' of schizophrenia, such as delusions of persecution, hearing voices or hallucinating, could be interpreted as a profoundly rational response to extremely disturbing experiences, such as growing up in a dysfunctional or damaging family environment.[3] The definition, causes and treatment of the 'psychoses' are still hotly debated, but that debate is beyond the scope of this book.

The more common and generally less severe forms of mental 'illness' are often referred to as the *neuroses*, and it is much less easy to fit these comfortably into the illness model. They include experiences such as depression, phobias (such as agoraphobia), anxiety and behaviours such as eating disorders or self-injury, some of which are so widespread as to be 'normal', and it is these which most commonly bring lesbians into contact with the mental health system. Some psychiatrists and other clinical practitioners insist that experiences such as depression are disorders of the brain caused by chemical imbalances and generally the result of a genetic predisposition. However, most people working in the mental health field now admit that there is no easy answer to the chicken-and-egg question: do chemical changes in the brain *cause* depression, anxiety, etc., or do these experiences *lead to* chemical changes in the brain, or do certain life experiences give rise to *both* alterations in mental state *and* changes in brain chemistry, with neither one causing the other? Whatever the relationship between brain chemistry and states such as depression and anxiety, there are reasons why lesbians may have a particularly difficult time of it when seeking help for such experiences.

Gender and insanity

The first problem is that we are women. Although men tend to outnumber women in diagnoses of psychosis, women hugely outnumber men when it comes to the so-called neuroses: especially depression, anxiety, eating disorders and phobias. Nobody has yet satisfactorily proved whether this means that women are *really* more likely to have these experiences than men, or whether the problem lies in diagnostic practices of the medical profession. It is certainly the case that, when presented with similar symptoms in male and female patients, doctors are more likely to assume that women's symptoms are psychological in origin and men's are physical (i.e., 'real').[4] It is also more acceptable for women to express 'weak' emotions such as fear or depression than it is for men to do so. Of course the second question is, if women really *do* suffer more from these experiences than men, what causes this?

Feminist researchers have identified many ways in which women are disadvantaged and discriminated against in the field of mental health, including the following.

- Our ideas of what is sane and insane are shaped by cultural beliefs about what is acceptable behaviour for men and for women. So behaviour which is considered normal for a man (like getting into a drunken fight in a pub) or for a woman (like crying at a romantic film) is likely to be interpreted as evidence of insanity if someone of the 'wrong' sex does it. Expressions of anger are especially likely to be interpreted as symptoms of mental illness in women. Clearly this has implications for lesbians, who may be consciously rebelling against a stereotypical female role.

- Generally accepted ideas about what constitutes a 'sane' person bear a marked resemblance to ideas about 'proper' adult masculine behaviour, whereas generally accepted ideas about what constitutes insanity or neurosis are remarkably similar to ideas about 'proper' adult female behaviour (Freud, for example, defined femininity as consisting of *passivity*, *masochism* and *narcissism*).[5] In other words, being a woman is *in itself* seen as akin to being neurotic. Lesbians are in a bit of a double bind here – if we accept a traditional female role we are neurotic because we are women, if we reject it we are neurotic because we cannot 'come to terms' with being female.

- The circumstances of many women's lives – including poverty, the isolation and stress of caring for small children, the double burden of paid work plus domestic labour – render women vulnerable to depression, anxiety and low self-esteem.[6] In addition to these stresses, homophobia and heterosexism take their toll on the self-esteem and wellbeing of lesbians.

- Although 'proper' feminine behaviour is seen as intrinsically neurotic, and although being obedient to traditional female gender roles is likely to cause intolerable stress, *rejecting* culturally accepted norms of feminine behaviour is seen as evidence of mental illness. Under this heading, 'symptoms' have included everything from failure to experience heterosexual desire to unwillingness to wear makeup.[7]

It doesn't take a great leap of the imagination to see that, as women who reject the bedrock of 'proper' female behaviour by desiring other women rather than men, lesbians risk being labelled mad by definition, and of course 'homosexuality' was defined as a mental illness until relatively recently, and is still classified as such in the *Manual of International Statistical Classification of Diseases, Injuries and Causes of Death*. However, it is unclear whether lesbians are more or less vulnerable than non-lesbian women to experiences such as depression and anxiety, since the substantial feminist literature on women and health contains very little material on lesbian mental health.

This neglect springs partly from the familiar tendency of non-lesbian feminists to ignore lesbians, but partly from the fact that the heterosexual female role is presented, in feminist accounts, as being at the root of many (non-lesbian) women's mental distress. The inability of men to be caring and empathetic, the isolation and exhaustion of caring for small children, the demands of what Lesley Doyal calls 'routine sex',[8] the low status of women in middle age, the identity crisis accompanying children leaving home – all these have been shown to make women vulnerable to depression and anxiety. What is more, this seems to be a cross-cultural phenomenon, affecting women in countries as far apart as India and Ecuador.[9]

Clearly, the traditional reproductive heterosexual relationship can make women mad. Yet, because researchers have not bothered to find out whether (or not) being a lesbian *protects* a woman from all this heterosexual torment, this is never said quite directly enough (perhaps the health promotion slogan 'Heterosexuality can damage your health' *is* hard to imagine . . .), and it is the 'female role', rather than the *heterosexual* female role, which is identified as damaging.

Researcher after researcher has conclusively demonstrated that heterosexuality is damaging to women's mental health.[10] However, few researchers have thought to investigate the ways in which *not* being a heterosexual woman affects the mental health of lesbians. Feminists have largely concentrated on demonstrating that the figure of the lesbian is used as an awful warning to police the behaviour of women in general. Jane Ussher is fairly typical of feminist writers on mental health when she comments that 'female sexuality outside the bounds of patriarchal control has always been deemed deviant',[11] but is also typical in that her brief passage on 'The Lesbian' refers to lesbians (along with spinsters and barren women) *only* as the psychiatric equivalent of witches. Her book on women and madness makes no attempt to discuss lesbians' experiences of madness or psychiatric care.

Mad with queer desires: homosexuality as mental illness

If lesbians have a difficult relationship to mental health because we are women, we have an additional set of difficulties because we are 'homosexual'. If simply being female is enough to label us neurotic, being queer is all too often seen as *in itself* a mental disorder. Most writers describing the historical relationship between lesbians (and gay men) and the mental health system agree that love, desire and sexual activity between members of the same sex was gradually absorbed into a *medical model* during the nineteenth and early twentieth centuries. In other words, homosexuality was seen not just as a symptom – *evidence* of existing mental illness or disturbance – but as an illness in its own right. This idea that homosexuality was an illness could not survive long within a scientific community that valued rationality and empirical, research-based evidence. It was challenged in 1969 by the Report of an American study funded by the National Institute of Mental Health and carried out by Dr Evelyn Hooker. Hooker's research demonstrated that there was no observable difference between the mental health and stability of heterosexual and homosexual individuals, and that psychologists and psychiatrists could not distinguish between heterosexuals and homosexuals on test results.[12] These findings were followed by many others in the same vein, and in response to such findings (and the energetic lobbying of lesbian and gay mental health professionals and activists) the American Psychiatric Association (APA) removed homosexuality from its official *Diagnostic and Statistical Manual of Mental Disorders* (DSM) in 1973. This step meant that lesbian and gay sexuality was officially no longer regarded as sick.

However, the story does not end here. As Richard Isay points out, different professions within the field of mental health continue to regard homosexuality as a sickness, the most important of which are psychoanalysts. 'Psychoanalysis,' he writes, 'in contrast to and in spite of [the] evidence, remains committed to the conviction that homosexuality is always pathological.'[13] Moreover, members of the APA have lobbied, unsuccessfully, to have homosexuality reinstated in the *DSM* as a mental illness and, as John Gonsiorek cautions, many continue to believe that it is an illness: 'The illness model of homosexuality is not dead; it is simply a minority opinion at this point in time'.[14] Indeed, the *Manual of International Statistical Classification of Diseases, Injuries and Causes of Death*, a diagnostic reference manual used by physicians around the world, *continues* to classify homosexuality as a mental illness.[15] This continuing disagreement has worrying consequences for lesbians seeking care from mental health practitioners. You may be lucky enough to find one who doesn't believe that being a lesbian means that you are sick, but you may just as well be stuck with one who does. Given the power that mental health professionals have, both over their clients and in shaping public opinion, this is troubling.

Moreover, the medical industry is a hugely profitable one, and commercial interests may have an influence on public opinion and on the beliefs of clinicians. In the 1960s the powerful Roche Laboratories published an advertising leaflet to promote their tranquillizers, in which they recommended these drugs in the 'treatment' of homosexuality. The leaflet asserted confidently that 'psychiatrists would probably agree unanimously on at least one point: the belief that the homosexual is a sick person'. Discussing this promotional exercise, Jeffrey Weeks points out that Roche were reflecting public opinion of the time: 'by 1965, 93 per cent of those polled in an opinion poll saw homosexuality as a form of illness requiring medical treatment'.[16] Proposing that homosexuality was a sickness that struck unwilling victims was, historically, a vital first step towards changing social attitudes and improving the social position of lesbians and gay men. But the consequences of the medical model were often serious for individuals. Many were subjected to 'treatments' for their 'illness' which ranged from the painful and unpleasant to the downright abusive. Even for the majority who were able to avoid such treatment by remaining firmly closeted, we can only guess at the damage done to their happiness and self-esteem by the belief that they were suffering from a mental illness.

Voices raised in protest: lesbian and gay affirmative practice

One of the important tasks of the lesbian and gay liberation movement was to repair the psychological damage done by centuries of abuse and, in particular, by decades of medicalizing same-sex love and desire. One key text from early on in the lesbian feminist movement makes this depressing statement:

Guilt is at the core of the Lesbian's life experience. It is her heritage from the past; it controls her present and robs her of her future. The dynamics of guilt pervade and order her days, draining her of her energy . . . the Lesbian withers under its influence or is forced to try to understand it – historically and personally – and vigorously to struggle free of it.[17]

This assertion, which reads very strangely from the newly assertive and confident position of today's younger lesbian, is a realistic recognition of the emotional and political work which needed to be done at the time. The book it is taken from, *Sappho was a Right-on Woman*, can be read as an extended exercise in developing self-esteem through consciousness-raising and political awareness. Such strategies were found throughout the new social movements of the

1960s and 1970s: Black Power, the women's movement, the anti-psychiatry movement and Gay Liberation. They were important in forming coherent groups strong enough and angry enough to get involved in political activism. In the context of homosexuality and the mental health establishment, such activism included 'zapping' mental health conferences, lobbying professional bodies and setting up lesbian- and gay-friendly alternatives to psychiatric clinics. Sidney Abbott and Barbara Love describe the work of one such, Identity House, which was set up in 1971 by 'a small group of professional therapists and members of Gay Liberation' and which aimed to provide services for lesbians and gay men which challenged the sickness model of homosexuality.[18] Such initiatives laid the foundation for the dramatic growth of the 'gay-affirmative' therapy movement, which is now one of the key elements of lesbian and gay communities in many industrialized nations.

There are many problems with gay-affirmative therapy. The work which they do is not based on adequate knowledge about lesbian mental health, simply because there has not been enough empirical research done. We simply do not know in enough detail how being a lesbian or living in a homophobic society affects your mental health, what mental health 'problems' are especially common among lesbians or how mental health services may best meet the needs of lesbian clients. This research is under way, but it is poorly funded and generally depends on the efforts of lesbian clinicians or researchers. Another problem is that therapists and others seem to feel the need to create a whole new diagnostic manual of neatly labelled syndromes or emotional disorders peculiar to lesbians (and to gay men). For example, there is widespread acceptance among many lesbians that lesbian relationships suffer uniquely from 'merger' (the idea being that the two women involved become unhealthily close, to the extent that they lose their sense of individual identity) or that we are prone to a terrifying disorder called 'lesbian bed death'.[19] Any theorist of sexuality worth her salt who does a cross-cultural comparison of these experiences with *heterosexual* couples would conclude in no time at all that there is nothing inherently lesbian about either of them. The trouble seems to be that the theorists who come up with these ideas have very little grasp of the research methodology which is needed, and they generalize from their work with lesbian clients without investigating how the same problem may be experienced in non-lesbian couples. This doesn't mean that there is anything inherently bad about lesbian researchers either, it is just that working in the kind of intellectual ghetto which seems to have been set up around the question of gay-affirmative therapy is not conducive to rigorous practice.

An additional problem with gay-affirmative practice is its close association with models of addiction growing out of the twelve-step alcoholism recovery programmes in the USA. The addiction model for what are loosely called dysfunctional human behaviours has expanded to incorporate not just recognized addictive substances like alcohol or opiates but behaviours that do not fit easily into a generally held understanding of addiction. You can now be addicted not only to food or stimulant drugs such as caffeine but to sex, to violence and even to love. What is more, if you are not an addict yourself you are almost certainly a co-addict or co-dependent. If being a lesbian is not pathological in itself, it increasingly feels as if many other behaviours are pathologized within lesbian communities. Perhaps, having grown up with a sickness model of our identity, we lesbians are simply unable to think of ourselves as anything other than sick?

This is not to reject the work of recovery programmes out of hand. There is no doubt that they have been invaluable for many distressed lesbians, and that for some they have meant the difference between life and death. Jane Futcher, for example, is rightly furious with lesbian academics who, with no personal experience of addiction and recovery, attack the recovery movement for supposedly distracting lesbians from political activism. She counters, 'in my case, being sober has fostered a desire and willingness to take responsibility, to become *more* politically active, to work for change and justice'.[20] Futcher herself is highly critical of Alcoholics Anonymous, which she describes as homophobic, sexist and racist. Nevertheless, it is clear from her account and that of other lesbians who have been helped by the recovery movement that it has been an important source of support to many. But it is important to locate behaviour such as addiction in its social context. For example, what sense does it make to talk of lesbians being 'addicted' to sex once you start to pick apart the complex threads which construct our lives and sexuality:

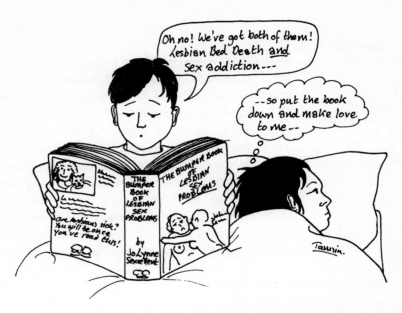

homophobia, the lack of support for long-term relationships, the powerful cultural association between lesbian identity and sexual performance and our need to reclaim a sense of sexual self-esteem in the face of the general belief that lesbianism is sick?

The final criticism of lesbian- and gay-affirmative therapies is that they exclude so many lesbians. Such therapies are almost exclusively located in the private sector and as such are too expensive for the majority of lesbians, who are less likely than gay men to be in well-paid jobs. Moreover, as Sophie Laws points out, 'someone who is too distressed to hold down a job would be unlikely to be able to pay for psychotherapy in any case'.[21] In addition to being beyond the means of many lesbians, gay-affirmative therapies have been criticized for being racist, classist and sexist,[22] and hence are unlikely to meet the needs of working-class or minority lesbians.

Today, any lesbian going through an emotional or psychological crisis has to confront both the misogyny and the homophobia of the mental health establishment and pick her way through the complex issues surrounding the services which may be available to her (if she can afford them) outside it. So, what can you do if you experience mental health problems, or if you are trying to support another lesbian with such problems?

Getting help

In a book this size it is not possible to address 'severe' mental illness properly. If you, or someone close to you, has been diagnosed with a severe and long-lasting condition such as schizophrenia or manic depression, get in touch with a mainstream mental health advocacy group such as MIND (see Further reading below). There is, however, much that may be done to prevent or to heal from those experiences commonly called 'minor mental illnesses' – although this term rather heartlessly trivializes what may be profoundly distressing experiences – including depression, anxiety (these two often go together) or phobias. There are also some strategies which may be useful for lesbians whose experiences include self-injury.

Falling into the black hole: depression and anxiety

Depression, often associated with anxiety, seems to be the commonest mental health problem experienced by women. Whether being a lesbian makes you more vulnerable to depression, protects you from depression or makes no difference is unclear. Since most heterosexual women's depression appears to stem either directly or indirectly from their heterosexuality, it might be supposed that being a lesbian makes you *less* vulnerable to depression. This supposition is borne out by a few accounts from women whose depressions vanished or became less severe when they made the transition from heterosexuality to lesbianism: 'Leaving home and loving women released me from the dead spell' writes Dorothy.[23] However, there are far more accounts detailing the damage which can be wreaked on a woman's self-esteem as she struggles to grow up and live as an adult lesbian in a society that hates and ridicules her, and it seems likely that this experience may lead to depression. There is so little research in this area that we cannot generalize one way or the other with any certainty. However, if you are depressed you will, quite frankly, not care much about research findings. You will want the experience to end. Understanding the reasons why you become depressed in the first place may help you out of it, and will certainly help you prevent it happening again, but when you are in a depression all that matters is finding your way out of an intolerable experience.

Depression affects different people in different ways. It is emphatically *not* the same thing as feeling miserable or 'down', even when miserable feelings persist over several days. Depression, which the medical profession distinguishes from simple unhappiness by refering to 'clinical depression', is a state which interferes with your ability to carry on with your usual life and may prevent you working, caring for yourself or your dependants or having any social life. You may experience any of a range of unpleasant physical symptoms: sickness or nausea, loss of appetite, difficulty sleeping, regularly waking very early in the morning, disturbances of digestion (constipation or diarrhoea), dizziness, headache, exhaustion, aching limbs, sore throat (with no obvious signs of infection), pains in the chest or stomach and physical weakness.

As if this were not enough, your mind can play strange games. You may become obsessed by upsetting or frightening thoughts, you may have nightmares, you may start to think about death or start to question the meaning of life, you may feel peculiarly unreal or disassociated from reality, you may even have some visual disturbances and you will almost certainly have trouble concentrating and may be unable to understand written or spoken language. These experiences may be very frightening, especially if you have not had them before. We tend to measure sanity against some notion of remaining articulate, rational and in control, and suddenly finding that you cannot even read a trashy novel or that you feel as if you don't exist can make you believe that you are really 'going mad'. Don't worry. Our ideas about what it means to 'go mad' are generally rather dramatic, formed of a heady mix of fictional characters (Mrs Rochester alone in her attic, Mrs Danvers smiling crazily as she burns to death in Manderley) and ill-informed beliefs about the 'psychotic episodes' experienced by a few seriously ill people. This kind of madness has little to do with depression, and you are *not* likely to go over some mythical edge separating the sane and the insane. Dealing with the miserable things that *are* happening to you will take up a lot of your energy, so don't make it worse by imagining total mental collapse!

Once you have got out the tunnel of depression once, the way your mind and body behaves when you are depressed may be familiar to you if you become depressed again. The trouble is, this familiarity can itself be frightening, since one characteristic of depression is that it is so overwhelming that the memory of non-depressed times in your life seem unreal, and it can start to feel as if the depressed you is the *real* you and anything else is just an illusion. At times like this the most helpful thing you (or anyone else) can do is to remind yourself that this *will pass*. It may take time, but time is the single most important healing factor in depression.

If you are one of the many people whose depression is mixed up with anxiety, you will know just how frightening fear itself can be. You may experience panic attacks during which your heart races, the blood seems to drain from your face and extremities, and you feel sick, faint, dizzy or suddenly drenched with sweat. You may feel desperately frantic, as if you have to run away, or you may have the sensation that you have dropped out of the world or that everything is closing in on you. Sounds may become very far away and muted, or may seem to overwhelm you. Sometimes such attacks are precipitated by a particular event – this is often what happens in phobias for example – but at other times they seem to strike at random and without warning. You may experience a more or less continual state of barely restrained terror, which makes it impossible to sleep, eat or function in your normal way, and the sensation of being tightly wound up like an overstretched wire may make you feel that you are about to 'snap' altogether.

There is much that you can do to alleviate anxiety, although depression itself is often more stubborn. If you are prone to anxiety you can prevent it by the following.

- *Get enough sleep and rest* – anxiety is often a sign of overwork and exhaustion.

- *Give up coffee* or, if you simply cannot face the idea, change to decaffeinated or cut down to one cup a day. Coffee is a powerful stimulant, and high levels of coffee consumption are enough to cause anxiety attacks in anyone. Even quite small amounts may spark off panic attacks in sensitive individuals.[24]

- *Eat properly*, avoiding processed or sugary foods which may contain additives that spark panic attacks, and eat plenty of fresh vegetables. Protein and cow's milk may have a calming effect (not much good if you are allergic), and most of us have 'comfort foods' which calm us, perhaps because of childhood associations.

- *Make use of naturally calming (legal) substances.* Some herbal teas, such as camomile, are very calming, and the scent of hops and lavendar have been used to calm agitated people for centuries. Try sleeping with a lavender bag under your pillow, or experiment with one of the range of 'natural' or herbal remedies for anxiety which are available in most chemist's shops.

- *Reduce your consumption of alcohol and nicotine.* Although the habit itself may reassure you (and the middle of a profound period of disturbance is not the best time to quit unless you have a great deal of support), the drugs themselves are not helpful in anxiety.

- *Exercise!* Physical exercise is a powerful tranquillizer and helps your body get rid of the adrenaline which is making you feel so panicky and buzzed out. It also releases endorphins, which make you feel good, and hence it helps lift depression. A quick run around the park, a few lengths of a swimming pool or a vigorous workout can make an almost miraculous difference to the way you feel. If you are too panicky to leave the house, try to get the use of a stationary exercise bike and pedal away when you feel anxious.

- *Relaxation exercises can help enormously*, although it can be very difficult to relax once you are in an anxious state. Because anxiety and stress are so common, there are relaxation classes in most towns and cities, and it can be very helpful to sign up for a course of lessons. Alternatively, try learning yoga, tai chi or meditation, all of which have evolved centuries of experience in calming and soothing anxiety.

> Prevention is better than cure, but even quite severe anxiety can be helped by these strategies. If you feel that your anxiety is so overwhelming or so severe that none of these techniques will help, do at least give them a go. Going to a doctor should be regarded as something to fall back on if these tried and tested self-help methods don't work, since doctors have very limited resources at their disposal.

If you seek medical help

If you do decide to ask your doctor for help in dealing with anxiety and/or depression, you may be advised to try the methods outlined above as a first step. More and more doctors are starting to suggest non-drug solutions to depression and anxiety, since they have (rightly) been criticized for handing out tranquillizers and anti-depressants much too readily, especially to women. However, the pharmaceuticals companies continue to market their drugs to doctors very aggressively, and 'new' anti-depressants or tranquillizers – such as Prozac – are often promoted to doctors as being non-addictive and free of the sorts of side-effects which were associated with older drugs. You may find that your doctor offers you drug treatment for your depression or anxiety, and this treatment may include sleeping pills, tranquillizers (anxiolytics, in trade terms) or anti-depressants. Remember that you don't have to take these drugs, but they have certainly been helpful to many people. Ironically, one of the consequences of concern about over-prescription of tranquillizers to women has been that some doctors are very unwilling to prescribe them, and there is concern that some women may be turning to cigarettes and alcohol instead.[25]

If you are prescribed a *psychotropic* (mood-altering) drug to help with depression or anxiety, and if you have not taken this drug before, it is a good idea to gather as much information as you can about how it works and what you may experience. When you are living through a period of depression or anxiety you will be highly sensitized to relatively insignificant changes in your thinking, mood and feelings, and it is important to be able to identify what is the 'illness' and what is the effects of the drug. Ideally, talk to someone who has taken the same drug. You can also get helpful information from the pharmacist who dispenses the prescription to you, from the doctor who prescribes it or from a mental health helpline or community group in your area. Anti-depressants in particular may be very difficult to take: they take several weeks to make any positive difference in your mood (your doctor should warn you of this) and they can make you feel stupified, unreal or nauseous, all of which may be very distressing if you are desperate just to feel normal again. However, if you do find tranquillizers, anti-depressants or sleeping pills helpful, they can offer an important contribution to relieving the unpleasant experiences of depression or anxiety for long enough to enable you to begin tackling what caused your depression in the first place.

Getting to the cause

Drugs, relaxation and lavender pillows can be very helpful in alleviating unpleasant sensations and experiences, but they cannot do anything about the cause of your miseries. Depression and anxiety are probably best thought of as your mind and body working together to tell you that there is something in your life that needs attention. Losses (whether recent or in the past), isolation, repressed anger, having to deal with an intolerable situation at work or at home, being worn down by stress or exhaustion, having been harmed emotionally or physically (for example, having been sexually abused or injured in an accident) – any or all of these may be the initial 'cause'. It can be very useful to put some energy into working out *why* you became depressed in the first place, and this is generally easiest to do with the help of a trained counsellor or therapist (see below).

Self-injury: a neglected experience

Self-injury can be a very distressing experience, both for individual lesbians who self-injure and for their friends, partners and family. Deliberate self-injury can range from pulling out hair to bruising, burning or (most commonly) cutting parts of your own body. It is important to distinguish between self-injury and attempted suicide, since they are not the same thing. Some people suggest that self-injury is part of a continuum of self-harm which ranges from indulging in pleasurable habits known to be harmful (such as drinking coffee or alcohol or using tobacco or street drugs) through obsessive harmful behaviours such as over-work or over-eating. However, there are very real differences between doing something which you know is harmful in the long term because it gives pleasure in the short term (such as smoking) and doing something which is both unpleasant and obviously harmful while you are doing it (such as cutting your arm). There are also differences between socially sanctioned forms of damaging behaviour (such as drinking too much alcohol or working too hard) and doing something which most people find shocking and incomprehensible. I am not sure how helpful it is to see self-injury in this way as part of a general 'package' of self-harmful behaviours.

Others, especially women who have personal experience of self-injury and who are working to support other women who self-injure, point out that self-injury is almost always experienced by the woman herself (and it is mostly women who self-injure) as a way of releasing terribly painful feelings. These feelings are often of badness, guilt or self-loathing, and there is growing evidence that for many women they may be linked to having been sexually abused.[26] There is no evidence that lesbians are more likely than non-lesbian women to self-injure, but there are certainly lesbians who do, and it is important that, if you are a lesbian who does, you are able to get what support you need. This means that lesbian communities need to become more aware of the issue.

It is important to distinguish between self-injury and sado-masochistic sex play. This is not to deny that there probably are some women whose behaviours might be classed as self-injury if they were not done within an erotic or fetishistic context. 'Sally', for example, associates her multiple genital piercings with periods of abuse in her life:

46 *There was a time in my life when I allowed myself to be manipulated by men, and some were quite violent. I acquired an addiction to pain, I'd need a painfix now and then and piercing became a safe way to achieve this. I no longer get pierced for this reason, but it helped wean me off my self-destructive habits.*[27] **99**

However, the accounts of women who self-injure do not support the idea that they are addicted to pain, and the majority of people (whether gay or not) who practise sadomasochism, piercing, bondage or fetishistic sex are clear that they do what they do for pleasure, not in response to psychological or emotional pain. It is disrespectful and unhelpful to them, and to women who self-injure, to see their actions as similar.

If you are a lesbian who self-injures you may feel isolated, scared or ashamed. You may find that others react to your self-injury with shock, horror or simple incomprehension, and fear of this reaction may lead you to conclude that you will not be able to find support in dealing with your self-injury. If you are a close friend or lover of a woman who self-injures, you may experience her behaviour as frightening, hard to understand or manipulative. Often self-injury can play a very destructive part in a relationship, since it can all too easily be used to punish or manipulate a partner: 'I felt so controlled by her cutting. I couldn't get angry, in case she cut herself. I felt she was punishing me . . . saying "look what you've made me do".'[28] On the other hand, a lesbian who does not self-injure may be tempted to label one who does as sick, out of control or dangerous.

The good news is that self-injury is beginning to be addressed in a much more positive way by health care workers, and there is a growing network of self-help groups and information services. Since most self-injury self-help networks have grown out of activism on the part of feminist mental health groups and women who have personal experience of self-injury, they are likely to be lesbian-positive and should be able to offer appropriate support for lesbians who want to stop self-injuring. A useful first step is to get hold of some of the publications listed in the Further Reading section. It is important to realize that self-injury is almost always a coping strategy, and that stopping will not help you unless you are able to understand why you have been doing it, and to get some support in working through some of those reasons and healing the inner hurts that led you to injure yourself in the first place. One of the first feminist groups to research the issue, Bristol Crisis Service for Women, offers this advice:

You are most likely to be able to stop your self-injury if you can understand and work on the issues in your life which underlie it. You need to develop other ways of coping with the things which hurting yourself has helped you to survive, and other ways of expressing the important things you want to say.[29]

Working in this way towards giving up self-injury obviously means that you have to find some kind of support, preferably from a trained counsellor or therapist or an established, well-facilitated, self-help group rather than relying on the goodwill of friends. This is true also for lesbians who are (or who tend to become) depressed or who experience anxiety states or phobias.

Talking about it: therapists and counsellors

There is a heated debate going on between some lesbian feminists, who insist that therapy is politically bad for lesbians, and others who believe that each of us has the right to use whatever is available that we find helpful. You may find yourself getting drawn into this argument if you decide to seek the services of a counsellor or therapist. Unfortunately, some lesbian communities seem to be happier to attack the choices of other lesbians than to challenge the homophobic insitutions of society which make our lives so difficult! Remember that you have the right to choose whatever support you need to get you through your life, and you do not have to defend your choices to appease anyone else's political sensitivities. Of course lesbians have to be critical and challenging of those aspects of the mental health system that perpetuate homophobia and cause hurt and damage to individual lesbians, but undermining other lesbians is not the best way to do this!

There are many different 'talk therapies' which you may find useful. These range from intensive, long-term work with a psychotherapist (which may involve several sessions a week over many years), through relatively short periods of weekly visits to a therapist or a set number of sessions with a counsellor. Counselling is probably the cheapest and easiest option to start with, since counsellors with basic training are often available through women's support groups, self-help groups or even some doctors' practices, and may be either very cheap or free. Counselling is supposed to be non-directive (they won't tell you what to do, just help you make sense of your experiences), and counsellors may have specialist training and experience in an area such as rape counselling, working with survivors of childhood abuse, or self-injury. Generally there is a limit to the number of sessions you are allocated (although some counsellors work in a more open-ended way) and, if you decide that the counselling has identified some areas of concern that you would like to go into more deeply, it might be worth considering moving on to therapy.

Some lesbians are very frightened that consulting their doctor with mental health problems may mean that they get referred to a psychiatrist. There are very good reasons for distrusting psychiatrists, who tend generally to have a very poor understanding of most women's lives, let alone of lesbian issues, but some lesbians have been helped by psychiatric treatment. 'Laura' writes: 'I consider my experience of the psychiatric world one of the luckiest breaks in my life', but cautions that 'the positive treatment I received is very, very rare in the public health service'.[30] Psychiatrists are no more homophobic and ignorant than the rest of the population. As Laura suggests, 'professionals in the psychiatric field are only human and often as frightened of looking at sexuality . . . as the vast majority of people',[31] but the difference between psychiatrists and other people is that they do have a lot of power, especially once you get into the mental health system. If you do decide to work with a psychiatrist, you will be entering a system that gives the psychiatrist a lot of power and disempowers you.

Therapy is a much more intensive experience than counselling, but much more in your control than psychiatry. However, lesbian or lesbian-friendly therapists may be hard to find, and therapy very seldom comes free. Some lesbian and/or feminist therapists offer a sliding scale but, nevertheless, you may be working with someone for a year or more, and this can end up being quite expensive. Therapists will often not work with people during a severe emotional or mental crisis, since you do need some basic emotional resilience to deal with the uncomfortable issues which can crop up during therapy sessions. You also, of course, need to be in the kind of job where you can get regular time off to go to your therapy, since most therapists keep office hours. So, however helpful it is (and many lesbians have found therapy very helpful indeed), it is likely to be out of reach of most of us. Alternatives to formal therapy may come into their own if therapy is out of the question. These include therapy groups or self-help groups focusing on a mental health issue, support groups or even telephone helplines.

Choosing what is right for you

When you are struggling to deal with an emotional or psychological crisis, it is far from easy to be thoughtful and critical about the kinds of service you want and need. At such times it can be invaluable to have the help and support of a friend who has personal experience of similar times of crisis, or to have access to a lesbian-friendly mental health service locally. As always, personal recommendation is the best guide to possibly useful services. A lesbian or lesbian-friendly doctor, therapist, counsellor or support group is not always easy to track down, and the personal experience of other lesbians is probably the most useful guide to local services you could have. If you don't have access to this kind of support, your first port of call should be your local lesbian and gay switchboard or help-line, or a mental health advocacy group.

In conclusion, we do not know enough about lesbian mental health issues because lesbians have been neglected in mental health research. We do, however, know enough about women's experiences of mental distress, and about the sorts of services that women have found useful, to be able to suggest what strategies are likely to be useful to lesbians. Sexuality is recognized as an important issue by most mental health activist groups and user organizations (although of course many heterosexual service users and ex-users are as homophobic as any other section of the population), and it is important for lesbian communities to recognize that mental health is an important issue for all of us. The strategies for preventing depression, anxiety and other very common distressing experiences are simple and often effective, but they cannot deal with the larger-scale *social* factors which have such important consequences for lesbians' mental health. Poverty, racism, homophobia and sexism start to damage us when they result in our having our children taken away, having to lead our loving relationships in secrecy and isolation, being unable to feed and care for ourselves and our families, being denied access to proper jobs, good health care or adequate housing or simply participating fully in our communities. Joan Busfield suggests that this may, in the long run, mean that treating mental health problems as an illness is not the answer:

individualising tendencies, which stem from the very nature of the clinical enterprise – healing individuals who are already sick – blind many of those involved in the care of people with mental disorders to the importance of the social and material conditions of individuals' lives that are often conducive to mental disorder.[32]

In other words, seeing someone as suffering from an illness may detract attention from what is really 'wrong' with their lives and the conditions they are struggling to live with. For lesbians, it is a cause for wonder and celebration that so many of us manage to live rich and generally contented lives in the teeth of a hostile society. It is no surprise whatsoever that so many of us go through periods of despair, psychological distress and misery. These issues belong in the open in lesbian communities, and we should take the lead in recognizing that 'mental health' is not a problem for a few individual lesbians but the concern of all of us.

Further reading

General

D. Davies (ed.), *Pink Therapy: A Therapist's Guide to Working with Lesbians and Gay Men* (Milton Keynes: Open University Press, 1996). Useful if you are looking for a therapist.

Boston Lesbian Psychologies Collective (eds), *Lesbian Psychologies: Explorations and Challenges* (London: University of Illinois Press, 1987).

Celia Kitzinger and Rachel Perkins, *Changing Our Minds* (London: Onlywomen Press, 1993). A lesbian feminist anti-therapy approach to lesbian mental health.

Kate Millet, *The Loony-Bin Trip* (London: Virago, 1990). Personal account of Millet's breakdowns and eventual withdrawal from drug treatment.

Bonnie Burstow, *Radical Feminist Therapy* (London: Sage, 1992).

A resource list on lesbians and mental health is available from the Lesbian Information Service, PO Box 8, Todmorden, Lancashire OL14 5TZ (tel.: 01706 817235). Send £4.50 to cover photocopying, post and packing.

In the USA, the National Women's Health Network has an information pack on depression. Send $7.50 to them at 514 10th Street, N.W., Ste 400, Washington DC 20004.

Self-help

Gerrilyn Smith and Kathy Nairne, *Dealing with Depression* (London: Women's Press, 1995 rev. edn).

Marny Hall, *The Lavender Couch: A Consumer's Guide to Psychotherapy for Lesbians and Gay Men* (Boston: Alyson, 1985). Self-help for self-injury.

Understanding Self Injury, *For Friends and Family* and *Self-help for Self Injury* (Bristol: Bristol Crisis Service for Women, 1994). Three lesbian-friendly booklets.

Good Practices in Mental Health, *Women and Mental Health: An Information Pack of Mental Health Services for Women in the United Kingdom* (London: Good Practices in Mental Health, 1994).

Networking

Bristol Crisis Service for Women,
PO Box 654, Bristol BS99 1XH
tel: 0117 925 1119

6 Growing Old Gracefully? Issues for Lesbians as We Age

By the time we reach late maturity, many of the problems which confronted us as younger lesbians have been resolved or have become less significant. We tend to have a stronger sense of self, to have evolved strategies for accepting or coming to terms with our sexuality or for surviving the homophobia of the wider society. A lifetime's experience has strengthened us and has taught us that we are able to survive life crises of various kinds. However, lesbians who today are in their sixties or above may have very different expectations and a much weaker sense of lesbian 'community' than lesbians who came out or grew up during the feminist resurgence of the 1960s and 1970s.

For years I lived next door to an elderly lesbian couple in a working-class area of Bristol. They were very traditionally butch and femme – Ellie was frequently mistaken for a man and Rose was a white-haired sweet old lady – and the street, where they had lived for forty-odd years, tacitly accepted them for who they were. When Rose was dying I spent as much time as possible with them, and when she had died I visited Ellie regularly. During those visits she finally plucked up the courage to say outright to me that she knew I was gay, and that 'You know how it was with me and Rose. We were gay too.' Then she said 'And that's the first time I've even said the word'. That, and the stories she told me and the photos she showed me about their time together, brought home to me how different it was for lesbians in those days. How much courage they had needed, and how invisible and unrecognized was her grief. It's not that people in the street were hostile, just that they were at a loss. It was amazing that I was around at that time, but it was no more than a lucky accident. I keep thinking of all the bereaved and lonely lesbians of that generation who don't happen to have confident 'out' younger lesbians move in next door to them at the right time. This is a generation who generally lack access to the support networks which many younger lesbians (though not all) take for granted. This is also a generation whose existence is not recognized by health and social care professionals. But age is not a problem for some 'other' group of lesbians. We are all growing older every day, and some of the things we do in our teens, twenties and thirties may have an impact on the kind of old age we can expect to enjoy.

Health in later life

There is no evidence whatsoever to suggest that lesbians face many specific *physical* problems as we get older. However, it is likely that the *implications* of the physical changes that come with ageing are different for lesbian and non-lesbian women, and there is no doubt that the *social* problems which confront older lesbians are very different from those confronting either younger lesbians or older non-lesbian women. Lesbians have less routine contact with the medical profession than non-lesbian women, since we have less need for contraceptive advice and aftercare and we are less willing to have regular cervical smears, so problems which may be picked up in heterosexually active women by routine examination may be missed in lesbians until they are advanced enough to cause symptoms.

Of course, this is not *necessarily* a disadvantage. For example the medical profession, encouraged by the pharmaceuticals industry, puts a considerable amount of pressure on women to accept hormone replacement therapy (HRT) for 'symptoms' of the menopause and to prevent osteoporosis. If lesbians see much less of our doctors, and if we have a critical and informed approach to gynaecology, we may be less likely to accept potentially harmful treatments of dubious benefit. However, there is a careful line to be walked between refusing suspect treatment from a well-informed position and failing to get necessary treatment because we do not trust doctors or simply because we are unaccustomed to the rituals of gynaecological care. This chapter aims to provide the basis for developing an informed approach to the health issues which can arise as we get older.

How do I know when I am 'old'?

The whole experience of getting older seems to be more fluid for lesbians than for non-lesbian women. Heterosexual women (and probably many bisexual women) are encouraged to value themselves according to their attractiveness to men, and heterosexual attractiveness for a woman means youth. In particular, many heterosexual women report that the experience of menopause is traumatic simply because they are forced to make a social and emotional transition from fertility into infertility. For many, this can feel as though their 'usefulness' is over. No longer able to produce children, how can they fit themselves into 'heterosexuality' when that heterosexuality is so firmly bound up with the production of offspring? In some cultures which mandate social roles for women which are narrow or restrictive relative to the white Anglo norm, this may be even more so. As Shivananda Kahn recently told a lesbian and gay health conference, 'Culturally, [South Asian] women do not have any sexuality. Her social role is that of "breeder"'.[1] For lesbians, who have a very different relationship to childbearing, this issue does not arise in the same way. As one lesbian put it:

Although I do have difficulty with ageing, I believe that it is easier as a lesbian. I am less self-conscious about cosmetic perfection, about weight gain and wrinkles – and feel that I have more sexual/romantic opportunities than a straight woman of my age.[2]

The question of when a woman is 'old' is not an easy one to answer. At a conference of old lesbians held at California State University in 1987, 'The 60 year olds thought 70 was old. The 70 year olds thought 80 was old. The 80 year olds thought 90 was old'.[3] Yet the sudden recognition that we really are getting older can dawn in our mid-thirties or forties. That moment when you are taking a long country walk and suddenly feel pain or stiffness in your joints and realize that it has become familiar without your noticing. The morning when you have to get up extra early to catch a train or plane, and the face that peers back at you from the bathroom mirror looks suddenly more like your grandmother than you. The amazed discovery of a grey hair or the faint first signs of 'liver spots' on the backs of your hands. The first time that a doctor or nurse says, casually, 'women of your age . . .' These moments herald for each of us the process of coming to terms with the fact that time is moving on and our bodies are already changing.

It is important, and gratifying, to know that relatively simple changes can reverse many health problems associated with ageing, and can prevent or delay the onset of others. By improving the way we treat our bodies, thirty-five- or forty-year-old lesbians can maintain a very good level of health and fitness and dramatically reduce the likelihood of problems such as osteoporosis or depression as they move into later life. On the other hand, gentle changes in diet or behaviour can sometimes improve the health of women in their nineties quite dramatically. The question to ask yourself is not, 'am I old yet?' but 'am I ready to recognize and deal with the fact that I am getting older *now*?' Just as it is never too late to make beneficial changes, so it is never too early to begin strengthening your body and planning your life to withstand the changes of age. Increasing the amount of fresh fruit and vegetables in your diet *at whatever age* reduces the likelihood of breast cancer or upper gastro-intestinal tract diseases as you age, whilst some estimates suggest that 'as much as *half* of the functional decline associated with ageing is the result of inactivity and can be reversed by exercise.'[4]

Such health-promoting changes are not all physical. We live in a society which places very little value on older people (especially women), which refuses to recognize that older lesbians exist at all and which pursues youth and beauty with hysterical determination. What is more, European, North American and Australasian societies are going through major demographic shifts which threaten the material wellbeing of their elderly citizens. Because of widespread improvements in living standards (and, to a lesser extent, medical care), people are living longer than ever before. It is only relatively recently that life expectancy in the so-called First World was similar to life expectancy in the so-called Third World today. In addition, people are having fewer children. This, combined with the worldwide recession which followed the oil crisis of the 1970s, means that the number of people who are economically active – in paid work – is shrinking at both ends (with fewer jobs available for school-leavers, and early retirement or redundancy common among mature workers), while the numbers of people who are economically dependent (the unemployed, the elderly, the chronically sick) are increasing. Thus, increasing numbers of people must somehow be supported with decreasing resources available.

The consequences of these changes have been especially disastrous for women.[5] Because of the heterosexual notion that male breadwinners are entitled to a 'family wage', whilst women need only 'pin money', women traditionally find themselves in part-time, insecure work which doesn't pay very well and fails to provide adequate pensions or sickness benefit. Elderly women, and women with responsibility for the care of others, are therefore likely to be living in poverty. 'The two poorest groups in the UK today are women raising children alone and women over sixty-five living alone.'[6]

It is less clear how this may affect lesbians. It is likely that lesbians who have been well served by the education system are better able than our non-lesbian sisters to develop and maintain a relatively well-paid and secure career. Some research suggests that because fewer of us take time out to look after children (the biggest single factor damaging women's earning potential and career path), and because we don't have to worry about emasculating our male partners by earning more than they do, or being seen as a ball-buster at work because we are promoted over male colleagues, we are more likely to do well at work,[7] and may end up with relatively good pensions. However, this is likely to hold good only for a minority of lesbians. The education system is likely to fail lesbians who are working-class, from some minority ethnic groups or who have physical or intellectual impairments. These women, the majority of lesbians, are far less likely to be in secure, pensionable employment.

The health consequences of poverty can be dire. Proper food, adequate clothing, a comfortable home, good heating and a supportive social network all become more important as we get older. Yet living in poverty makes it extremely difficult to achieve these necessary things. This is why it is so important not to put off thinking about the consequences of ageing. In our thirties, forties and fifties we are better able to plan our lives so that we can avoid or minimize poverty and isolation in later life. For lesbians who find themselves struggling with poverty in later years, the question becomes how to prioritize our limited spending so that we can best support our own health and wellbeing. The advice in Chapter 2 will help in maintaining good basic health, but there are health issues of particular relevance to older lesbians which are dealt with here.

Menopause: a non-medical approach

There is no need to be scared of the menopause. Indeed, recent research suggests that lesbians may experience their menopause in a much more positive way than our non-lesbian sisters:

> the lesbians surveyed and interviewed do seem, in general, to have a positive attitude about menopause and aging. They do seem to be less subject than heterosexual women to the wrath of ageism and partner expectations. They do not seem to descend so deeply into ageist and sexist despair, even when the issues . . . are the same . . . lesbians at menopause seem to be completely free from the fear that their partners will no longer find them attractive.[8]

However, there is a scarcity of information about the menopause for lesbians, and this in itself can give rise to anxiety and uncertainty. Lee Lynch recounts an experience common to lesbians trying to find relevant information about menopause:

> The more books I read, the more tired I became of reading about child-bearing years being over and about husbands finding wives unattractive and the wives, heaven forbid, drying up and destroying marital bliss. Where were the lesbian stories? It's not that I thought menopause would be physically different for lesbians, but I certainly didn't find myself in the words I was reading.[9]

Some of the physical experiences of menopause can be overwhelming or difficult to manage for some women. Menopause, like any other bodily change, cannot be seen as 'just' a physical or biological event; it comes with all sorts of complex meanings for women, and those meanings have social and psychological consequences. Menopause is also loaded with cultural meanings about what it means to be a woman, and about sexuality. *Of course* menopause is going to be different for lesbians!

It may be helpful to summarize the basic information about the experiences that may be associated with menopause for many lesbians. Despite the alarmist tendencies of the medical profession to make menopause sound like a deficiency disease, it is neither an illness nor a biological emergency but a normal life change, just like puberty. There are three signs of bodily change which may accompany the menopause: your periods stop, you may experience some changes to your vagina and/or you may get the (in)famous 'hot flushes' ('flashes' in North America). It is perhaps not surprising that the menopause has been largely ignored by medical researchers and does not play a major role in basic medical training, so many doctors have very little idea of what is 'normal' for a woman at this time. What we do know is that the *only* experience shared by all women during their menopause is that menstrual bleeding stops. This may be quite sudden: your period may simply not start when you expect it to, and you may never get another one. It is more likely that they will become irregular, either much further apart than is usual for you, or (and this can be less easy to deal with) much closer together. They may become lighter or heavier, and you may get pre-menstrual signs which are new for you, such as breast tenderness or irritability.

Although doctors tend to assume that any menstrual changes in a woman over forty are due to the menopause, there are other possible causes for such changes, including diabetes, gall bladder disease or high blood pressure (hypertension). A good doctor will test for other possible causes, or will do a simple test to establish the level of hormones in your blood, before assuming that your experiences are attributable to the menopause. These tests are not foolproof, but can be useful, so if you don't get offered them, ask. Once you are reasonably certain that you are going through your menopause, you can begin taking steps to ensure that it is a trouble-free and positive experience. After all, just imagine . . . no more period pains, no more spending money on towels or tampons, no more ethical dilemmas about disposal, no more headaches, cramps, mood swings . . . freedom!

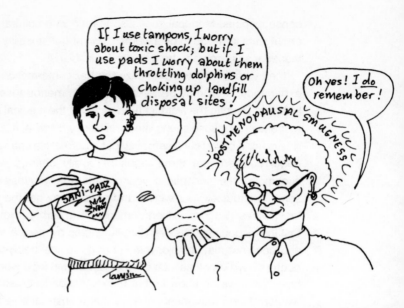

Many of my heterosexual women friends are haunted by the spectre of the 'dry vagina'. This seems to be a potent symbol of the sexual and relationship problems which they fear in the context of their relationships with men. Lesbians, whose sexual practices do not necessarily depend on penetration, who spend much longer on lovemaking than heterosexuals[10] and whose sexual encounters are not so rigidly structured, do not spend hours anxiously debating the terrors of the dry vagina. Nevertheless, the tissues lining the vagina do become drier and more fragile after menopause for most women, and it is a good idea to experiment with vaginal lubricants such as KY Jelly, Crisco or Glyde if the kind of sex you enjoy becomes more difficult.

Hot flushes are reported by between 47 per cent and 85 per cent of women, depending on which survey you read.[11] A minority of women find them very unpleasant, but they do not bother all women who experience them. In one large survey only 15.5 per cent of the women surveyed reported finding them a problem. Whether or not you find them difficult seems to depend on how you interpret them, and on how those around you react. The sensation of a hot flush is not in itself unpleasant. In fact, some lesbians have said that they experience them as mildly pleasant or sensual. If you are the sort of woman who needs to feel in control of your body, and who resists or dislikes physical experiences out of your control, you are more likely to find hot flushes unpleasant.

What exactly *is* a hot flush? For many women, it is no more than a brief sensation of increased warmth, for others it may be a wave of heat accompanied by sudden profuse sweating, for still others it begins with a chilled sensation, similar to the onset of a cold or flu.

Sometime during my forty-ninth year, I wake in the night to feel a line of fire creeping up from my midsection, over my chest, and into my face. Aha! I think. This must be a hot flash. I find that recognition somehow satisfying.[12]

For most women, as the feeling of heat fades it is at least sometimes followed by a sensation of cold. Other signs which may be linked with hot flushes for some women include blushing over the face, neck and chest, feelings of anxiety or nausea, and increased heart rate or palpitations. This is a bit of a Catch-22 situation, since women who are not troubled by them tend not to experience these other signs. What we don't know is whether such signs as anxiety and palpitations are caused by an emotional reaction to the flush, or whether women who have these experiences react negatively to hot flushes *because* of them. What is certain is that if you can relax and accept what is happening to your body, rather than thinking 'Oh no! Here comes a hot flush!', you will not be sending alarm signals to your body and are less likely to feel anxious, panicky or nauseous.

Helpful strategies for dealing with hot flushes

Women have reported that all the following are useful in minimizing the nuisance of hot flushes.

- *Reduce alcohol intake*: alcohol dilates blood vessels and can exacerbate the sensation of heat.

- *Get into the habit of dressing in layers*, so that you can easily respond to a temporary increase in body heat by taking off your cardigan or jacket, then your sweatshirt or waistcoat, and have a cool shirt, blouse or T-shirt as a final layer. Being in control of your body temperature is made much easier.

- *Breathe slowly, calmly and deeply* if the flush makes you feel anxious. Try saying to yourself, 'Mmmmmm . . . what a lovely warm feeling!' rather than 'Oh no, here we go again!'

- *Take your bath or shower a degree or two cooler than usual*, to avoid bumping up your body temperature.

- *Where possible, sit near a window that you can open*, carry a fan with you or step outside for a few minutes' fresh air when you have a flush.

Many lesbians report that, rather than being an unpleasant nuisance, flushes can be fun, an opportunity to pay caring attention to yourself or the signal for a few minutes' relaxation. There are other positive approaches as well:

It was a freezing December night when I lay in bed, dreading to get up and go down a long cold hall to an even colder bathroom. Then I had a hot flush, and, all of a sudden, it was very easy to leave my warm bed![13]

Unpleasant menopausal experiences

Apart from hot flushes, missed periods and changes in the vagina, other signs associated with the menopause include irritability and/or depression and heavy bleeding. These more directly unpleasant experiences are not inevitable, and are reported by a minority of women. Nevertheless, they can be very dispiriting.

Heavy bleeding can be inconvenient – sometimes it is so heavy that normal tampons or towels have to be changed many times a day – distressing and exhausting. It can result in anaemia (iron deficiency in the blood), extreme fatigue and physical weakness. If it happens to you, it is important to discuss it with your doctor or other health adviser, as fibroids or other problems in the uterus could be to blame. Your doctor will probably give you a full gynaecological examination (see Chapter 9 for some idea of what this involves) and may decide to do a 'scrape' or a D&C (dilation and curettage).[14] You may then be prescribed a hormonal treatment to control the bleeding. If this happens, ask your doctor how long s/he envisages that you will have to take the hormones. Taken over a few months in order to relieve heavy bleeding, hormone treatments (such as the mini-pill or combined pill) can be extremely useful. However, if your doctor anticipates that you will need to take this medication for more than a few months, or if s/he wants to put you on hormone replacement therapy (HRT), you will need to think very carefully about the implications. You may find it useful to read the section on HRT that follows in the discussion of osteoporosis, and you should certainly make use of the Further reading section to get as much advice as possible if you are considering HRT to control heavy bleeding.

Depression, anxiety and tension are reported by a significant minority of women during their menopause. If you have experienced hormone-related mood swings during your menstrual cycle or during pregnancy, the signs will feel very familiar. The difference is that the cycle will shift, and a few women find that they become depressed or anxious for several weeks or months. There is a tendency among the medical profession for depression and anxiety around the time of the menopause to be labelled a menopausal 'symptom', whereas of course it is equally possible that it has other causes. If you are experiencing such a profound depression that you feel you really cannot handle it, or if you are really having a hard time with anxiety, read the section on depression and anxiety in Chapter 5 on mental health. It helps to remember that any mood changes which accompany your menopause are unlikely to last very long, and that your mood *will* lighten as time passes and your body adjusts.

Dem dry bones! Osteoporosis

After decades of neglect, osteoporosis is receiving a lot of attention from the medical profession and the media. It is probably cynical of me to suspect that this has a lot to do with the publicity campaigns of the drugs industry, which profits by promoting HRT as a means of preventing or 'curing' osteoporosis.[15] Osteoporosis affects far more women than men (it is not unknown among men, although relatively rare), and describes a condition where the bones begin to lose mass and density, to weaken and become brittle, to the point where they may start to crumble at the joints or become very vulnerable to fractures. The resultant damage can be very disabling, since the bones of the spine, the knee and hip joints and bones in the hands and wrists may be affected, resulting in restricted activity or mobility. Osteoporosis is caused by a reduction in the production of new bone tissue; it is closely related to the amount of calcium present in our bodies, and to the ability of our bodies to absorb and make use of this calcium.

The good news is that osteoporosis is relatively easy to prevent, and you don't need to take medication or calcium supplements to do so. There are two main steps which any lesbian, whatever her age, can take to reduce the likelihood of developing osteoporosis, or to limit its effects. The first is to maintain a good intake of calcium in your diet. Calcium is found in dairy produce, especially whole milk, as well as in greens, parsley, spinach, broccoli, tinned sardines or salmon (with the bones), brazil nuts, corn products such as tortillas and (if you are feeling flush!) 'real' ice creams such as Häagen Dazs or Ben and Jerry's. The easiest source throughout a lifetime is whole milk. Many of us have started drinking low-fat or skimmed milk in an effort to reduce our fat intake, but whole milk is only about three per cent fat, and you can drink two or three glasses a day without worrying about cholesterol. If you cannot tolerate cow's milk, make sure you drink calcium-enriched soya milk, or compensate by increasing your intake of oily canned fish or green vegetables.

The second important strategy is putting your bones to work and stimulating them to increase mass and density. In order to do this, you have to take the kind of exercise which puts gentle and continuous stress on the bones, and the best ways of doing this are weight training and swimming. Weight training need not be done in gymnasiums with complex equipment (although this is increasingly popular among lesbians of all ages and can be great fun). It can simply mean doing gentle exercise such as running on the spot, skipping or step-exercising with special light weights attached to your wrists and ankles, or carrying your shopping in carefully balanced shopping bags as you walk back from the shops. If you have limited mobility, a physiotherapist will be able to teach you an appropriate exercise routine using weights to strengthen your bones.

Maintaining mental alertness

There are many myths surrounding old age, and one of the most frightening is the automatic association of ageing with mental decay, confusion and dementia. In fact, current research suggests that intellectual capacity remains remarkably stable throughout life and, if exercised and stimulated, some mental functions actually *improve* in later years. There are three main ways in which our thinking may degenerate as we age. Confusion, forgetfulness and slow thinking can be caused at any age by depression, isolation and lack of stimulation. They may also be caused by what the medical profession calls *benign senescent forgetfulness*, a decline in memory caused by changes that take place in the brain as we age. Finally, there are diseases and disorders which can lead to mental confusion. The best known of these is probably Alzheimer's disease, but there are others, such as multi-infarct dementia, a condition caused by repeated small strokes affecting the brain tissues. As well as these three key factors, some impairment in mental function may be caused by malnutrition, by conditions such as AIDS or diabetes, or by prescription or over-the-counter drugs, especially in combination. Careful and attentive diagnosis is required to pinpoint the cause of mental confusion or forgetfulness in older lesbians.

There is nothing special about the structure of lesbian brains which would make stroke, dementia or Alzheimer's either more or less likely. However, the isolation, loneliness and poverty experienced by many elderly lesbians *is* likely to put them at greater risk of depression and malnutrition. We know absolutely nothing about the long-term social and psychological consequences of living in a homophobic society, but they are likely to be damaging to mental health and intellectual function. In addition, the *consequences* of forgetfulness or confusion may be very different for lesbians than for non-lesbian women. Lesbians who are over sixty now are less likely than younger lesbians to have had children, and so will have less access to family support and care as they age. They are less likely to have developed frank and trusting relationships with health care professionals or to have access to voluntary support or lesbian community networks, and are more likely to have broken ties with their extended families of origin. Elderly lesbians who need residential care, home nursing or hospital care are unlikely to be offered services which recognize and respect their needs as lesbians. Lesbians who are confused, forgetful or dementing may be terrified that they will inadvertently reveal their sexual orientation in an unsafe context and be punished or mistreated in consequence.

Strategies for coping with forgetfulness

All of us become forgetful under stress or when fatigued. For many women this means most of our lives, and for lesbians there is no doubt that the additional stresses of concealing our sexuality or dealing with the consequences of *refusing* concealment will take their toll on memory and intellectual alertness at times. If you are experiencing difficulty with short-term memory it does not mean that you have taken the first steps on the road to full dementia. By all means seek professional advice if you are worried, but remember that most causes of memory lapse are temporary. Whatever the reasons for your memory lapses, you may find the following strategies helpful.

- *Create a 'memory corner' in your home.* This is the place where you automatically put essential items like your keys, spectacles, diary, handbag, pension book, medication, etc. It can be a drawer, shelf, box or table. If you always put essential items in your memory corner, you should never have to waste time and energy panicking about losing them. Once it becomes a habit, you won't even have to remember to put things there.

- If you have problems with names, *keep a photograph album* with pictures of your friends, family and work colleagues clearly labelled with their names. If you have to remember birthdays, simply put their date of birth under each one's picture. Then at the beginning of each month, go through the album and make a note of that month's birthdays on your calendar.

- *Keep a notebook or diary on you at all times* and write down any arrangements and appointments you make *when you make them*. This includes appointments with doctors and dentists, dates to have coffee or meals with friends, etc. You can also use this book to make lists of things you have to do each day, shopping to be done, etc. If you use a book rather than odd bits of paper you won't find that you have lost the list when you need it. A spiral-bound notebook is especially useful, since you can tear pages out when you no longer need them.

- *Organize medication to be taken during each week* by using an ice-cube tray or egg box marked with days of the week. Keep it by your bed and check it each morning and night. You will know you have taken your medication if the compartment for the day is empty. If you have trouble knowing what day it is, get into the habit of listening to the news on a radio station which tells you the day and date, and cross each day off on a calendar at bedtime each day.

- *Try to talk to people as often as possible.* Memory is linked to speech and language use, and anyone who spends long periods of time without talking to other people can become withdrawn and confused. If you live alone and do not have many visitors, pass the time of day with shop assistants or bus drivers, join a voluntary group or arrange to attend a local day care or drop-in centre, or get in touch with your local lesbian or lesbian and gay helpline. If you are able to get hold of lesbian and gay magazines or newsletters, write a letter to the editor asking if anyone would be interested in setting up a discussion or social group for older lesbians in your area. Such groups are increasingly common, and may have a lot to offer you.

- *Drink less alcohol,* and ask the advice of your local pharmacist or druggist about any medications you are taking. Even over-the-counter medications for colds or digestive upsets may react badly with other medication to affect your memory.

If you, or someone close to you, is diagnosed as suffering from memory loss or confusion caused by a clinical condition which is progressive – such as Alzheimer's disease or HIV-related dementia – remember that some such diseases are treatable, and that the effects of others may be significantly reduced with appropriate help and support. Get in touch with a help-line or support group and find out what is on offer.

General health issues in ageing

As we age, it becomes even more important to pay attention to our wellbeing, and this is as true of lesbians as of anyone else. Because of the shameful history of homophobia in the health and social care professions, lesbians are less likely to seek health care when we need to. This may be especially true for older lesbians who have not been involved in the more assertive, activist culture of younger lesbians and who are more fearful and less confident in their dealings with professionals. It is also the case that old age is not regarded positively in Euro-American cultures, and that many who work in the caring professions hold very stereotyped or dismissive beliefs about ageing. Additionally, as much feminist research has shown with devastating clarity, the male-dominated health care industry is riddled with sexism and largely ignorant about many social and medical issues which affect women. As lesbians age, we may be exposed to threefold disadvantage in our relationships with our health and social care providers, who may be ignorant of our needs – because we are women, because we are ageing and because we are lesbians.

In this context, the new consumerist approach to health care, although politically troubling in many ways, offers an opportunity for change. As the numbers of elderly people increase, elders will become a force to be reckoned with, and it is more likely that appropriate services will be provided if users demand them. Now is perhaps the time to start getting stroppy!

The key issues in general health and wellbeing as we age are our feet, our dental and oral health, our weight and strength, our cardiovascular system and (especially for lesbians) our sexuality and body-image. If you make use of the information in previous chapters on good eating and exercise, you should be able to maintain the health of your heart and lungs, to avoid lugging around too much body weight and to be positive about your level of fitness. Feet, teeth, body-image, strength and sexuality may need particular care.

Feet

Our feet are of great importance to wellbeing. They are the foundation of our mobility, and are likely to suffer from a variety of aches, pains and disorders after a lifetime's use (and, quite likely, abuse!). Yet we tend to neglect them until it is too late. One benefit of being a lesbian is that *perhaps* we are less likely to have spent decades tottering down the street in ridiculous fashion footwear which deforms the tendons, muscles and bones of the foot. Whisper a word of thanks for Birkenstocks, trainers and Doc Martens, for sensible flatties and men's shoes! Yet very few people reach a ripe old age having paid loving attention to their feet over the years. If you suffer from foot pain, callouses, corns, bunions, hammer toes, ingrowing toenails or whatever, make it a priority to seek professional advice and care. If this is not available on the NHS or not covered by your insurance plan, make enquiries of your local complementary practitioners. Reflexology, therapeutic massage and aromatherapy can all help with some foot disorders, and you may be able to negotiate special rates if you are living on a low income.

The best approach to foot problems, as with anything else, is prevention. Keep feet clean, cut toenails regularly, wear shoes which are the right size, comfortable, supportive and warm. Shoes are generally a very expensive item of clothing but, if it is at all possible to save up for a good pair, do so. They should outlast cheap shoes, and will help prevent foot problems which may lead in the end to restricted mobility, pain and expensive treatments. Trainers are quite good for you in one way – because they are 'cushioned' they absorb the impact of walking on tarmac and concrete surfaces and reduce damage to the ankle, knee and hip. However, waterproof ones may be expensive, and all of them tend to make the feet sweat, which can lead to problems such as athlete's foot. If you can afford it, it may be a good idea to wear trainers in the warmer months but they are not a good all-weather shoe.

It is highly pleasurable and beneficial to give your feet a massage once a week. If you can reach your feet, it will help keep you supple as well as helping your feet. If you cannot, it may be worth *gently* trying to do so until you have regained some suppleness and can. If touching your feet is difficult, *do not* attempt to do so standing up. Sit on a sofa, or put your feet up in front of your armchair on a footstool. If you use a wheelchair, or have no movement in your legs or arms, get a friend to massage your feet and legs once or twice a week. Even if you cannot feel it, it will improve circulation of blood and lymph fluid in your legs and feet. When massaging feet, use a little baby oil, massage oil or olive oil. You don't need much, and it is often pleasant to soak your feet first in warm water. This may be done in the bath, or in a plastic washing-up bowl. If you use a bowl, half fill it and lay a clean towel underneath it so that you can simply move your feet from the bowl to rest them on the towel.

Oral health

Our mouths are more than just our teeth! Unlike previous generations, lesbians ageing now are likely to have many of their natural teeth remaining. It is worth putting some effort into keeping them, since dentures (however good) are nothing like as effective as real teeth, and the major dentistry involved in operations like capping and crowning can be expensive and painful. Anecdotal evidence may suggest that toothless lesbians find new ways to increase their expertise in giving their partners pleasure through oral sex but, even if this is the case, it is at the cost of comfort and variety in eating! Teeth are more often lost through gum disease than through tooth decay, though you can reduce the risk of decay by cutting down on sugary foods and drinks, chewing sugar-free gum after meals (this stimulates saliva, which rinses plaque from the teeth) and using a fluoride mouthwash. The information given on healthy eating above (Chapter 2) will also enable you to eat in a way which reduces damage to your teeth. An adequate intake of vitamins is essential to keeping your mouth healthy, and ulcers or a sore mouth or tongue are classic warning signs of vitamin deficiency. Gum disease can be prevented by regular brushing, flossing every day and getting regular dental health check-ups. I am not aware of any research on lesbian dental health, but the fact that most dentists are men is likely to be at least one factor discouraging many of us from seeking dental treatment.[16] There is also evidence that fear of expense puts many older people off visiting their dentist regularly, and elderly lesbians are more likely to be living in poverty than their heterosexual counterparts. You may qualify for free NHS treatment, or your dentist may offer reduced fees for older patients. If not, you can budget for an annual or six-monthly check-up, much as you budget for telephone or gas bills, if you ask your dentist in advance how much s/he will charge for a check-up, and try to fit it into your financial planning. Many people who take out health insurance do not bother with dental insurance, which need not be expensive and may be well worth considering if you have enough financial leeway.

Weight and strength

It is important as we age not to carry too much excess weight around, but also not to be too thin! Elderly people who are very thin are more at risk from hypothermia, and tend to take longer to recover from illness or hospital treatment. Those who are very fat may have joint problems, or may be more at risk (although the jury is still out on this one) of heart disease and respiratory problems. We also tend to need less food as we age, indeed it has been suggested that maintaining our regular intake of food past the age of fifty to fifty-five will result in a weight gain of a pound a year.[17] Not exactly drastic, but worth knowing nevertheless.

Whatever your weight, age or mobility, maintaining strength is important. The section above on osteoporosis suggests ways of maintaining or increasing strength in muscles and bones, but you also need to make sure your diet contains enough protein and that you are able to get enough rest and sleep. Exercise which develops muscle strength actually increases the amount of muscle fibre, and this process takes place up to thirty-six hours *after* you have done the exercise. Your body needs to be at rest for this muscle-building to happen, so it is actually counter-productive to weight train or do strengthening exercises every day, since you will miss out on this essential period of rest.

Sexuality and body-image

The pressure to stay 'young and beautiful' which haunts non-lesbian women and gay men is certainly less extreme for lesbians, and there is evidence to support the belief that, as we age, lesbians continue to enjoy passionate and satisfying sexual relationships and encounters in a more relaxed way than non-lesbian women.[18] Our culture, especially where it has been touched by feminism, is more vocally appreciative of the qualities of older women, and may be more accepting of great age differences in partnerships:

When I was sixty-five I fell in love with a woman who was twenty-three years younger than I was . . . This was the most complete relationship of my life. It was romantic, passionate, sharing, intellectual. It was everything I had read about but never exerienced – such fullness and balance.[19]

Nevertheless, the most highly visible section of the lesbian community consists of young women, and, although there has been a dramatic increase in the number of lesbians portrayed in film and in the press and broadcast media, they are almost exclusively young and attractive. There is an increasingly active and vocal movement of older lesbians, insisting that the wider lesbian communities should recognize that ageism does exist among lesbians and that older lesbians cannot be dismissed as asexual, past it or not worth paying attention to.[20] In some minority communities, such as some Asian communities in Britain, Koori or Maori communities in Australia/New Zealand, or African/British and African/American communities, there is a tradition of respecting and valuing elders, but homophobia within these communities may make this respect inaccessible to their older lesbian members.

One of the central issues for lesbians as we age, and as the number of lesbians who are undeniably younger than us increases, is how we feel about our bodies, and the consequences of that for our sexuality. We live in cultures where the sexuality of old people is denied or dismissed, and where attractiveness – especially for women – is remorselessly linked to youth. The cosmetics, pharmaceutical and medical industries spend huge sums of money encouraging the idea that you are sexually attractive *only* if your face and body do not show the signs of ageing. Creams, potions and operations promise to conceal or eradicate lines, wrinkles and sagging skin, and there are dyes and wigs to conceal thinning or greying hair. So our first feeling when we look in the mirror and see wrinkles or grey hair, or when we touch our arm or neck absentmindedly and feel loose skin, may be one of panic or grief.

The process of coming to terms with the inevitable changes that accompany ageing is one which each of us must go through at her own time and in her own way. It is, however, cheering to know that older lesbians seem to have more sex, report more satisfaction with their sex lives and are more likely to be having sex even when not in a relationship, than older non-lesbian women.[21] Again, it is probably true that what helps here is transforming your approach. If you spend time paying attention to the ways in which time is changing your body, and to how you feel about it, rather than looking away and pretending it isn't happening, you are more likely to experience those changes as neutral or beneficial rather than frightening. Of course it would be foolish to deny that fear *is* inevitably associated with these changes. They may alert us to our mortality, make us feel that time is running out or remind us that the old are devalued in our society.

Get together with friends of your own age and discuss what you are experiencing. If you feel that your life is speeding by and the feeling scares you, it is probably a sign that you have things left undone which are important for you to do – some unfinished business with partners, children, families or friends, an ambition not yet realized, a dream endlessly put off. If you have always wanted to go hang-gliding, learn to play an instrument, make love in a moving train or write your autobiography, perhaps now is the time to do it. If your life is full of meaning and offers you the kind of stimulus and nourishment that you need, you are more likely to welcome the signs of ageing as the visible marks of a well- and fully lived life. If your life seems empty and lacking in achievement, it really *is* never too late.

Conclusion

Although there are some painful problems confronting lesbians who grew up in the first half of the twentieth century and whose lives have been lived largely under stressful conditions of secrecy and fear, there are many things to celebrate about being a lesbian as we age. It is true that many of the things necessary to wellbeing and good health cost money, and that older lesbians are more likely to be living in poverty than our gay brothers. For many ageing lesbians, isolation and the neglect of the health and social care professions pose very real and stubborn problems. Yet it is never too early to make the sorts of changes which can result in a healthier and more pleasurable old age, and it is never too late to make our lives richer and our bodies stronger and fitter. As lesbians, we do have many advantages; it takes a lot of guts to survive as a lesbian in a society which is casually hostile, and that means that we can all be stubborn and more assertive when required. We are accustomed to dealing with the knowledge that we disgust and frighten lots of people, so becoming a disgusting and frightening old person may come as less of a shock! We may also be less constrained by the demands of femininity than our non-lesbian sisters, and may be more independent, more assertive and less damaged by a lifetime conforming to shifting fashion norms. A growing number of old lesbians are coming together to make the sorts of changes, both in their lesbian communities and in mainstream society, that they want to see. And now, when the issue of lesbian health is just beginning to receive attention from health and social care professionals, is the best time to insist that they should recognize and meet the needs of elderly lesbians. For ageing lesbians, the prospect may be far from easy, but it is certainly better than it ever has been.

Further reading

Lee Lynch and Akia Woods (eds), *Off the Rag: Lesbians Writing on Menopause* (Norwich, Vermont: New Victoria Publishers,1996). I can't recommend this one too highly. Lesbians of every kind relating what menopause has meant to them. Rush out and buy it!

Barbara Sang, Joyce Warshow and Adrienne Smith, *Lesbians at Midlife: The Creative Transition* (San Francisco: Spinsters, 1991).

Dena Taylor, Sumrall Taylor and Amber Coverdale (eds), *Women of the Fourteenth Moon: Writings on Menopause* (Boston: Crossing Press, 1991).

Jean Shapiro, (US edition by Paula Brown Doress and Diana Laskin Siegal), *Ourselves, Growing Older: Women Ageing with Knowledge and Power* (London: Fontana, 1989). The best and most comprehensive resource on ageing for women, including lesbians.

Suzanne Neild and Rosalind Pearson (eds), *Women Like Us* (London: Women's Press, 1992). Life stories of older lesbians from the pre-Stonewall generation.

Barbara Macdonald with Cynthia Rich, *Look Me in the Eye: Old Women, Aging and Ageism* (London: Women's Press, 1984). Writings on ageing by politically astute lesbian couple.

7 Chronic Illness and Disability

Most of us live for at least most of the time with the (comforting) illusion that there is a clear division between wellness and illness, and between disabled and non-disabled people. In fact, things are not so simple. Short-term acute episodes of illness or injury, such as a dose of flu or a sprained ankle, are experienced as blocks of time, periods in our lives during which we were (temporarily) ill but which we can leave behind us once we are fully recovered. However, it is not so easy to 'leave behind' the long-term consequences of even a straightforward injury such as a broken bone if it leaves us with recurring pain (perhaps a tendency to ache during long walks or during cold weather) or if it gives rise to indirect damage (perhaps trapped or damaged nerves or some permanent weakness in the site of injury). Probably most adults experience some form of reduction or damage to their physical, emotional or intellectual abilities, from shortsightedness to migraines, from a fear of crowds, spiders or snakes to an allergic reaction of some kind. Very many women carry the long-term consequences of childhood abuse or sexual violence, all of which may be experienced as very disabling. Moreover, very few people get to the end of their lifetime *without* experiencing some sensory impairment, reduction in mobility or other damaged intellectual or physical function. None of us is any more than *temporarily* able-bodied, few of us are 'severely' able-bodied (i.e., having perfect function in body and mind), and chronic ill health or impairment can (and do) happen to anyone at any time. So having some understanding of the implications of chronic illness or impairment for lesbians is important for us all. Only a tiny minority of lesbians will travel from cradle to grave without having to deal with the consequences of chronic and/or disabling conditions, whether for ourselves or for our lovers, friends or communities.

At the same time, however, it is important to recognize that there are significant differences between various experiences of disability. Being born with a severe impairment of sensory function (blindness, deafness) or mobility (having little or no sensation or function in one or more limbs, or having problems with motor control, etc.) is a very different thing from acquiring such impairments in later life. It is useful to remember that bodily and mental perfection are unrealistic goals, not a norm, and that there is no fixed cut-off point between 'the disabled' and 'the able-bodied'. However, it is just as offensive to ignore the realities of disability as it is to ignore the realities of homophobia. Wearing glasses is not the same as being blind, and having experience of exhaustion does not mean that you know just what it is like to have ME.[1] After all, no lesbian would accept a straight woman's claim that she understood all about homophobia because she kissed her best friend at junior school.

It is also important to recognize that disability is not a biological condition but a social one. It is not the physical or intellectual *impairment* that directly restricts an individual's ability to enjoy a productive and full life, rather it is the failure of societies to recognize and provide for the specific needs of people with impairments. Being dependent on glasses to correct poor vision is not generally thought of as disabling in industrial societies, but it most certainly is where glasses, contact lenses and corrective laser surgery are not available. Similarly, using a wheelchair is disabling *only* when the design of pavements, public transport, homes, workplaces and public buildings does not take wheelchair users into consideration. As Susan Lonsdale concludes:

Having a physical disability means living in society as a minority group whose particular needs are not adequately recognized or taken into account, and whose different appearance often leads to being treated differently and less equally [sic]. *This usually means being at greater risk of poverty and exclusion.*[2]

Since living as a lesbian shares many of these penalties, it is clear that lesbians with impairments are likely to be doubly disabled.

What is special about the lesbian experience?

Because our societies generally believe that chronic illness and disability are things which happen to individuals at the level of physical, biological damage, there is very little understanding of how or why they may have particular implications for lesbians. Certainly there is no evidence that chronic illnesses or impairment are more likely to happen to lesbians,[3] but, when they do, their impact may be very different for lesbians and non-lesbians. It is likely that, for lesbians, the experience of chronic illness or disability will be made more stressful or difficult in at least four key areas.

- Having a chronic illness or impairment means that you are likely to be coming into frequent contact with a variety of health care, social care or rehabilitation services. This may pose particular problems to do with how safe it is to come out to service providers, and how to ensure that your needs for information and support are met and that partners and lesbian friends are treated with respect.

- Being ill or disabled from an early age may mean that young lesbians – especially those who spend time in institutional settings – are isolated not only from other lesbians and lesbian communities but perhaps even from an awareness that lesbians exist. Becoming chronically ill or disabled in adult life means forging very different links to your lesbian peers and community.

- Having a chronic illness or disability, from whatever age, may have a profound effect on your sexuality and on the kinds of sexual activities you enjoy or the nature of the sexual relationships you want and are able to establish. This will also impact on your lover(s) and on the relationships between you.

- All of the above, combined with the social emphasis on bodily perfection and a narrow ideal of beauty, may result in deep-seated changes to your sense of yourself as a lesbian. You may need, or be pushed, to adopt an identity as a sick or disabled person which may take the place of your lesbian identity, or may conflict with it.

Any or all of these difficult issues may have to be worked through with little or no support, since one of the key features of being chronically ill or disabled is isolation. However, there may also be very real advantages in facing illness or disability as a lesbian. We are less likely to be faced with the terrors of being 'unmarriageable', as described by one feminist writer:

Young women, suffering from chronic sickness, disability or deformity, have to face the additional social disadvantage of being regarded as less valuable and desirable on the 'marriage market'. Many personal accounts by young disabled girls include the cry: 'Who will want to marry me?'[4]

Moreover, lesbian communities may be more supportive of women with chronic illness and impairments, as one disabled lesbian suggests: 'Being a lesbian and part of the feminist community has made coping with my disability somewhat easier . . . the growing community awareness of disabled rights is refreshing and helpful.'[5] As lesbians, we are all accustomed to dealing with stigma on a daily basis, which should (at least in theory) mean that lesbian communities are better able to recognize, understand and challenge the stigma associated with disability and chronic illness. However, these advantages may seem insignificant when set against the daily experience of dealing with impairment and disability. This chapter explores some of the issues which chronic illness and impairment may raise for lesbians, and suggests strategies for dealing with them. I cannot stress too strongly, however, that disability is not a personal struggle. It must not be left to individual lesbians and their partners and friends to 'cope' with. It is in the interests of all lesbians that these issues are confronted within and by lesbian communities, and lesbians should work together with the disability rights movement to that end. This is also a very under-researched area, so I would encourage any lesbians in a position to carry out this kind of research to get on down and do it!

When does sickness become chronic become impairment?

It is helpful at this point to discuss some of the differences and similarities between various experiences of being disabled. You may have a long-lasting debilitating illness which is unlikely to be permanent (such as ME), a long-lasting illness which may or may not become permanent (such as rheumatoid arthritis) or an illness that you know to be permanent (such as lupus or emphysema), that may or may not be progressive. You may be born with an impairment which is progressive (such as muscular dystrophy) or one which is not progressive (such as weak or absent limbs), or you may, as a result of injury, acquire an impairment (such as an amputated limb or paralysis resulting from spinal injury), which may or may not lead to progressive deterioration or indirectly related damage. Whether you are chronically ill or have a specific impairment, you may experience your condition as predictable or wildly unpredictable, which may have important consequences for your ability to 'manage' and organize your life. There are also specific difficulties facing women who have an invisible condition (such as epilepsy) or one whose reality is questioned (like environmental allergies or ME). Finally, you may be living with an illness or condition which is likely to cause your death in the longer or shorter term. All these factors will influence how you live your life on both a practical and emotional level, and will have a greater or lesser impact on your sense of self, your relationships with those close to you, your ability and desire to work and your involvement in your lesbian community and other communities important to you.

Interactions with health professionals: lots and often!

Whether an impairment is something we are born with or something that happens to us later in life, it almost inevitably means frequent contact with health professionals. This is an issue for all chronically sick or disabled people, since the medical profession is (understandably) motivated by the desire to make things better, and what a doctor understands by 'better' may be very different from what the client or patient wants (or, in many cases, can afford). This desire to make things better has different consequences depending on where you live. In Britain, where treatment in the National Health Service is free, endless interventions may be made – in the form of surgery, wonder drugs or the latest developments in physiotherapy – in order to achieve sometimes tiny 'improvements'. Faced with a chronic condition which is not responsive to known treatments, new and experimental therapies may be tried over and over again. This may be exactly what you want and need if you have decided to invest your energies into a battle against your illness or impairment. Unfortunately, medical treatments have side effects, and being on the receiving end of this kind of well-intentioned experimentation may be as troublesome as the condition itself. It is also emotionally exhausting to have your hopes raised over and over again by fruitless attempts to make you 'better'. However, the days when patients were expected to be the passive and grateful recipients of medical attention are passing and, although some consultants do still seem to believe that they are minor gods, the majority are nowadays far better equipped to form good working relationships with their clients and to pay some attention to their wishes.

For anyone living in a country where health care is still closely linked to ability to pay, the idea of limitless medical attention may seem utopian. When you are unable to access the surgery, drugs or physiotherapy that you need because your insurance doesn't cover it or you don't have the money, it leaves a very bitter taste in the mouth. This is something which may be particularly devastating for lesbians, since employment-related health care benefits or insurance policies are unlikely to cover same-sex partners or the non-biological children of same-sex partnerships.

Whatever the financial issues, the relationship between you and the medical profession is likely to be influenced by your being a lesbian. All disabled or chronically sick people face a contradiction in their dealings with health care workers; being a 'good patient' demands that you behave in a childlike manner, obedient to the instructions of staff, quiet and submissive and generally good humoured, but dealing with the implications of chronic illness or impairment demands that you be assertive and strong. For lesbians, this contradiction may be particularly painful. As lesbians we are obliged to defend ourselves against the homophobia of our wider society, and this is likely to be especially important when we are vulnerable, ill or in pain. Some of us evolve coping strategies which are assertive, forthright and strong: I'm a lesbian, I'm happy this way and if you have a problem with that, it's your problem, not mine. Others rely on concealment, taking advantage of the general assumption that all women are heterosexual to pass as straight and avoid conflict, or take care to behave politely, reasonably and with gentleness in order to deflect hostility or to challenge homophobic assumptions about lesbians as man-hating troublemakers. Whichever strategy we adopt (and most of us use a range of different approaches for different situations) in our need to protect ourselves against the homophobia we may meet in our contact with health care professionals, the conflict between the docility of the 'good patient' and the strength of the 'heroic' disabled woman struggling against the odds is likely to be a particularly difficult one for lesbians.

For lesbians who have partners, there is an added dimension to interactions with health care systems. In some cases a partner may be able to share the burden of such interactions, helping to ensure that your wishes are met, that you are both given as much information as you need to continue making informed decisions about your care and generally acting as advocate and ally. However, the extent to which this is possible depends on the extent to which your relationship is recognized by staff. It is probably a good idea to be open and assertive about this from the very beginning, although you will have to use your own judgement here. If you have reason to believe that coming out as a couple will be risky, there is no sense in doing so. True, your bravery may well make it easier for the next lesbian couple to gain acceptance in that environment, but your first responsibility is to your own wellbeing and your relationship. The lesbian nation is not known for handing out medals for heroism in the face of the enemy under such circumstances! However, do not assume that health care workers are inevitably anti-lesbian. A fair proportion of medical and nursing professionals are themselves lesbian or gay, and it is becoming easier in some places for them to be out at work and therefore to be supportive to you. Although medicine is an especially conservative profession, and nurses in particular may hold stringent religious beliefs which conflict with their duty to provide good-quality care to lesbians, things are slowly changing. Increasingly, lesbians who need long-term medical care are reporting good experiences with clinical, nursing and paramedical staff.

Questions of identity

A lesbian identity is a strange thing, forged out of necessity. If those who hold power in society did not condemn the love, desire and sexual pleasures shared between people of the same sex and if women were not subordinate to men, then preferring women to men would be no more significant than preferring cats to dogs, or milk chocolate to bitter. As it is, the simple choice to act on our desires for women has profound consequences in almost every part of our lives. Heterosexual people don't build an identity around their sexuality; they have no need to, since heterosex is just assumed to be normal, natural and right. It isn't what heterosexuals do, it is just what *people* do. Lesbians and gay men, on the other hand, have to build our identities and our communities around what we do in bed which, when you think about it, is a fairly fragile foundation. What is more, our communities are often closely interwoven with our sense of lesbian identity, since it is from other lesbians that we get the affirmation and positive feedback that is usually denied us by our families of origin and wider cultures. As lesbian psychotherapist Sarah Pearlman writes, 'This sense of community helps make bearable the rejection and contempt present in the larger world'.[6]

There are many problems with lesbian identity and lesbian community for lesbians who are or who become chronically ill or disabled. Chronic illness and disability can be very isolating experiences. This can be due to their physical or emotional consequences: if you are easily exhausted, physically frail, in pain or emotionally fragile it may simply not be possible for you to attend lesbian social or political events, get to community meeting places or participate in networking. It may even be difficult to tolerate friends visiting. If this is your experience, there are strategies which you may find helpful in maintaining some kind of contact with other lesbians and reaffirming your sense of yourself as a lesbian. If you want visits, letters, audiotapes or telephone calls from lesbian friends, ask someone to ring round your friends and tell them exactly what you want. If you are new to an area and want this sort of contact in order to make links with whatever lesbian community is out there, get someone to find out whether there is a local lesbian newsletter, community bookshop, café, bar or women's centre. Get a letter in the newsletter or a card on the noticeboard at the women's centre, introducing yourself and describing the kind of contact you are looking for. Be as clear as possible. You may be interested in meeting a possible sex partner or future lover, or simply want someone to read to you, help with shopping or drop in for a cup of coffee. If you can cope only with short visits, make this clear from the start; it is not a good basis for a friendship if you are wretchedly longing for your well-meaning visitor to leave but are too polite or too exhausted to say so!

It is not only the direct consequences of illness or impairment that can lead to isolation. Although lesbian communities are more aware of disability issues than many other groups, there is still a lack of truly accessible venues. Lesbians as a group tend to be poor and have few resources, so it is far from easy to make the kinds of changes in environment or facilities which would improve the access or support available to disabled lesbians. Local lesbian communities vary enormously in the resources they can draw upon. A large city in the USA may support a thriving lesbian micro-culture with food shops, bookshops, meeting rooms, cafés and restaurants as well as bars and clubs, although such enterprises may depend on attracting some non-lesbian customers for economic survival. In a small town in England or an isolated village in Scotland there may well be no facilities for lesbians at all. In such circumstances a 'local lesbian community' may be no more than a group of five or six women who meet at each other's houses. Obviously it is easier for a large urban community to provide a range of accessible events and facilities.

It should not be the responsibility of lesbians who are disabled or chronically ill to demand that their local lesbian community recognizes their needs. However, in the real world this is all too often what happens, just as it is lesbians who have to insist that the needs of lesbians are recognized in mixed lesbian and gay environments or

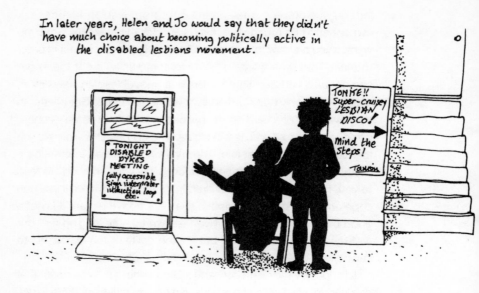

In later years, Helen and Jo would say that they didn't have much choice about becoming politically active in the disabled lesbians movement.

in the mainstream. It may be frustrating, enraging or scary to find that lesbians 'out there' seem to have no awareness of or interest in including you, and it can be tempting to just give up and retreat. It is in these circumstances that a disabled lesbians group can offer the best support. One disabled lesbian writes:

The disabled lesbian group has let me hang out with my disability, to touch it in different ways, to understand myself through touch. To understand through sharing our differences and our similarities . . . Being a lesbian is very hard for me right now.[7]

Your local switchboard should be able to give you information about any disabled lesbians' groups in your area, and in Britain social services should have this information as well. If there is no group, you may be able to get one going. This need not require you to take responsibility for organizing or leading a group, just putting the word about on the grapevine and getting a few people to meet up at someone's house. There may be help available in setting up or running a disabled lesbians' group, either from social services or from voluntary groups or charities. Check it out.

Sex, lovers and all that jazz

Most chronic illnesses and impairments can affect our sexuality. The disability rights movement has made great strides in getting disabled people recognized as sexual people with the same rights to a satisfying sex life as anyone, but there is still a long way to go. In particular, there is still little recognition of the sexual needs of disabled women, and rehabilitation efforts are largely directed at men. This is largely the result of historical accident: 'rehabilitation itself grew out of a concern for the war disabled, most of whom have always been male. This . . . has led to a service in which the involvement of women is inhibited.'[8] Combine the tendency to focus on the needs of men with a determination to ignore the troublesome issue of sex, and you have a situation where disabled women are deprived of the most basic information and support about sex. As Susan Lonsdale concludes, 'This attitude is manifested in the lack of information that there is available for disabled women on sexual activity, contraception and childbirth'.[9] As Lonsdale's own approach makes all too clear, if the needs of heterosexual women are neglected, even feminist writers tend to ignore the existence of disabled lesbians entirely.

Many lesbians recognize the brief moment of panic which can descend at the end of a relationship with a lover; if I am not having sex with another woman, does that mean I am not a lesbian? Since our lesbian identity is defined by our sexual relationships, it can be hard to find confidence in ourselves as lesbians if we are not in a sexual relationship, or if we are in a relationship where sex is infrequent or unimportant. The consequences of illness and disability can hit hard at our sexual lives and relationships, making it harder for us to have sex in certain ways or to have orgasms, to meet lovers or to work at maintaining long-term sexual contact with our partners. These consequences are not the same for all disabled lesbians. To be born with an impairment may mean that you have had to work hard to build a sense of yourself as a sexual person and a lesbian, especially if you have spent much time in institutional settings where there is seldom much privacy or opportunity for sexual exploration. Disabled women who spend much time in segregated institutions are even more likely than other women to have been sexually abused or exploited, and it can be extremely difficult to get the appropriate support to heal the scars of such abuse. In such circumstances it is unhelpful that many people seem to regard lesbianism as a safe option for women who are too disabled or too traumatized to manage 'real' relationships with men: 'Lesbianism', writes Lonsdale, 'is an important option for some women, and it often offers supportive and less threatening relationships than those with men.'[10] Many lesbians will recognize this as an all-too-familiar heterosexual fantasy that conveniently ignores both the strength of lesbian passion and the realities of homophobia!

Women who become disabled or chronically ill later in life face the trauma, denial and hard work of accepting their changed lives, altered bodies and new selves. There is a very real sense in which this requires us to forge a new identity built to a greater or lesser extent on our disablement, a process which can be extremely painful:

Sometimes it gets hard to separate my first life from my second life: quad life. I keep thinking how I'd like to stand up and walk away to a shower, wash away my night-sweat, drown the intrusive memories. But I'm a quad now. An eleven-year-old quad. We don't let the first life hurt us at this age. I have a position and an identity to reflect.[11]

Just as other identities – Jewish, black, mother, etc. – may conflict with our lesbian identity, so too may an identity as a disabled person. Connections to and bonds with other disabled people may feel much stronger and more important than our connection with able-bodied lesbians. And this conflict may have an impact on our relationships with our lovers, as well as with our lesbian communities.

If complex identity issues, and the losses and desexualization of disability in this disabling society put stresses on our relationships, so too do the direct consequences of illness and disability. Lesbian sex is generally a more thoughtful, protracted and egalitarian business than heterosex.[12] Lesbians just can't get away with lying back and thinking of England for ten minutes. You have to have the energy and ability to receive pleasure, *and* the energy and ability to give it. Even a common disabling injury such as Repetitive Strain Injury (RSI), which may seem relatively trivial, can have a dramatic effect on lesbian sexual activity. Sophie, a lesbian with RSI, is explicit about its effects on her relationship with her lover:

It's misery, and the effect on sex is obvious. Those sexy rough and tumbles sort of lose their tension when you can't give as good as you get and it's a foregone conclusion who's gonna go under. Fucking can be painful too. Fear of causing more damage can make both the sufferer and her lover(s) cautious and inhibited, so RSI doesn't just strain the hands, it can put a lot of strain on relationships as well.[13]

These concerns apply to many other chronic conditions as well as to RSI. Fortunately, sex between two women can take a variety of forms, and there is much that may be done to reduce the strain on an injured body part. Your lover can take pleasure from your body in any number of ways without requiring much in the way of hard work from you. She can press and rub her clitoris against any part of you that is appropriate, clothed or unclothed, as you lie on a bed or firm surface, sit on a sofa or in a wheelchair, or even stand. Oral sex is possible in many positions too. With you lying on your back she can kneel over your face so that you can lick, kiss and suck her clitoris, or she can lie on a (strong enough!) table, propped up with cushions if necessary, and you can lick her while sitting in a chair or wheelchair. If she likes penetration, you can buy dildos of all shapes and sizes from lesbian mail order suppliers (check the small ads in your local gay press), and these may be strapped to your thigh, knee, arm or pelvis. If you cannot afford a harness, or if you do not like the feel of leather, cut a small slit in a stocking or a pair of tights and poke the dildo through that (it is best to cut a much smaller hole than you think you will need, or the wretched thing will come unstuck at a crucial moment), before using the rest of the stocking/tights to tie it in place. Be careful not to cut off the blood supply if you attach it to a part of yourself which has limited sensation. If you are likely to use your home-made harness regularly it makes sense to sew velcro strips on to it so that you can attach and release it easily.

Whatever strategies you evolve to widen your erotic possibilities, do remember to develop a matching sexual care and cleanliness routine. If you have limited sensation and/or mobility you will already know your own degree of vulnerability to unnoticed bruises or infections, but your usual caution may be thrown to the winds during sex, and a new partner may need you to alert her to possible areas where extra care from her will be needed.

If you have limited sensation in your genital area, or no sensation at all, it is well worth spending time exploring other pleasurable sensations. 'There is some evidence', writes Susan Lonsdale, 'of women discovering new erogenous zones after disability [sic], with heightened sensations in those parts of their body not affected by the disability.'[14] This is one area where there are likely to be important differences between women whose impairment was present from birth or early childhood and those who become disabled after they have become familiar with their able-bodied sexual responses. Whichever applies to you, don't let anyone else tell you what you do or do not experience sexually, or attempt to define your pleasures for you. Even women who have lost their clitoris as a result of genital mutilation (euphemistically called 'female circumcision') sometimes report that they have orgasms.[15] Such findings do not make sense within the bio-medical model of female sexual response, which just goes to show that bio-medicine can be a pretty inadequate way of understanding sexuality!

If you have little or no sensation in your vagina or vulva, penetration is something that needs to be done carefully. There is no law which says that you should not experiment with penetration, and you may find that it can give pleasurable sensations, or that it is emotionally important to you. However, it is easy to damage sensitive tissue if you cannot feel pain, and there may be a risk of minor injury to your urethra or cervix. In such circumstances inanimate objects such as dildos need to be used with extreme care, and are probably best avoided altogether. Fingers (your own or your lover's) can move with gentleness and sensitivity or with quite powerful force while their owner remains alert to the possibility of bruising. You may wish to explore the possibilities of anal penetration, in which case the same precautions apply with added emphasis, since the vagina is considerably more robust than the rectum. If you have unreliable sensation in your pelvic area you should *not* attempt anal penetration with any inanimate object, since any damage in the rectum or lower bowel may have potentially serious consequences.

However, there is much more to sex than simple physical technique. Some illnesses and impairments can cause extreme exhaustion, debility or physical weakness, and these can mean that we just don't feel up to having sex, or that it is frustratingly difficult to reach orgasm. In these circumstances, it may be easier to give your partner pleasure than to take pleasure yourself. It may be enough for both of you if you are able to hold her close while she masturbates or if you can strap a dildo to your thigh and leave the energetic effort up to her. However, if you do go beyond your physical limits, there may be a price to pay in terms of future pain or exhaustion, or a build up of resentment. Morag, a lesbian doctor who has ME, writes:

Of course sex is affected too. There are times when my hand and arm are screaming at me to stop, while she's groaning her way to an orgasm. The orgasm usually wins, but I'm left with a weak, painful arm for hours afterwards.[16]

It helps to recognize that, although sex is an important and central part in lesbian relationships and in our sense of ourselves as lesbians, the problems which illness or disability may introduce into our sex lives are really no different from the problems which they introduce to the rest of our lives together. If you have managed to successfully negotiate problems in other areas, there is no reason why you should not be as successful in bed. On the other hand, there is more to having a good relationship than good sex. Lesbians who are chronically sick or disabled do have the right to expect their lovers to recognize the impact that this has on *all* aspects of their lives together. Gilly, a lesbian who is recovering from ME, was interviewed for this book:

❝ *I started a relationship with a woman who was a rock climber and super-fit. She would swim forty lengths of the pool or run a few miles before breakfast and she had a training schedule in her diary for each week. I explained that I wasn't fully recovered from my ME, but she was quite unable to understand that I really could not stay up til eleven every night, wake up before six to have breakfast with her and go on eight-mile walks across steep, rough terrain. The sex was fine but the rest of the relationship wasn't, and four months after we got together I was spending days in bed again, exhausted.* ❞

Paying attention to the whole relationship rather than seeing the sex in isolation is the key to building and maintaining a successful partnership, and this is just as true for couples dealing with a chronic illness or disability.

Disabled lesbians share many of the experiences of disabled non-lesbians, and it may be easier to get understanding and support from the disabled community than from the lesbian community. However, lesbian communities may make greater efforts to be accessible to disabled members than non-lesbian communities, and the disability rights movement can be very heterosexist. There may be times when this feels like a no-win situation – it's not OK to be a lesbian in the context of disability and it's not OK to be disabled in a lesbian context – but there are important benefits to be gained from both communities. The continuing task is for a lesbian-friendly disability movement, for a disability-aware lesbian community and for strong links to be forged between the two movements in the shared fight for full human rights and social transformation.

Further reading

Susan E. Browne, Debra Connors and Nanci Stern (eds), *With the Power of Each Breath: A Disabled Women's Anthology* (San Francisco: Cleis Press, 1985). Personal accounts from women, many of whom are lesbians, dealing with a range of disabilities.

Judith Barrington (ed.), *An Intimate Wilderness: Lesbian Writers on Sexuality* (Portland, Oregon: Eighth Mountain Press, 1991). Contains accounts from disabled and chronically sick women.

Kirsten Hearn, 'Oi! What About Us?' in Bob Cant and Susan Hemmings (eds), *Radical Records: Thirty Years of Lesbian and Gay History* (London: Routledge, 1988). Getting disability issues on the lesbian and gay agenda.

Tom Shakespeare, Kath Gillespie-Sells and Dominic Davies, *The Sexual Politics of Disability* (London: Cassell, 1996). Contains a lot of gay and lesbian material.

Michael Oliver, *The Politics of Disablement* (London: Macmillan, 1990). Good on disability politics, but not on lesbian (or gay) issues.

Susan Lonsdale, *Women and Disability: The Experience of Physical Disability Among Women* (London: Macmillan, 1990). A useful introduction to some of the key issues, but Lonsdale really misses the point about lesbians!

Kath Gillespie-Sells and David Ruebain, *Disability OUT* (London: Channel 4 Television, 1992). Informative booklet published to accompany a network programme about lesbians and gay men with disabilities. You can get a copy by writing to: OUT – DISABILITY, PO Box 4000, London W3 6XJ, or Cardiff CF5 2XT. It is free, but send a stamped, self-addressed A4 envelope.

On sex for disabled lesbians

Pat Califia, *Sapphistry: The Book of Lesbian Sexuality* (Tallahassee: Naiad, 1988). Much of this book is useful and there is a more substantial chunk on disability than can be found in most lesbian sex guides.

Jill Lessing, 'Sex and Disability' in JoAnn Loulan, *Lesbian Sex* (San Francisco: Spinsters Ink, 1984). Also useful.

8 Far to Travel: Dying and Grieving

It is often said that being born and dying are the only experiences common to all human beings. Yet in Western societies we have developed a way of dealing with death which, far from acknowledging its inevitability, makes it seem extraordinary, catastrophic and private. As faith in religion has been replaced by faith in scientific medicine, death has come to be seen as a failure rather than as the natural end of all of us. Medical science has no concept of an afterlife, and the inevitable consequence of this is that our death can be seen only as an ending rather than as the next stage in the journey of a spirit or soul. Of course there are advantages in accepting that this life is all you get; one way in which organized religion has always maintained the political status quo is by getting people to concentrate on their own immortal souls (which would be put in peril by anything so sinful as rebellion against those in power) rather than on improving the conditions of life here on earth. Lesbians have little cause for loyalty to the powerful religions of the world, all of which promote deeply negative views of women and same-sex love. However, giving up belief in survival after death has a high emotional and psychological cost. It is against all instinct to believe that you will one day simply cease to be. Indeed for many people it continues to be a psychological impossibility to accept this about themselves or those they love. Moreover, many millions of people who are adherents of the dominant religions (i.e., the majority of the world's population) continue to subscribe to doctrines which claim that death is not a final end. Nevertheless, even those who can find comfort in religious faith have grown up in a world where Western scientific medicine dominates the field of health and illness, and the religious approach to dying comes into conflict with the medicalized view of death as something that should be prevented at all costs.

These changes in cultural approaches to death have, in the industrialized West, combined with rapid improvements in public health and in the provision of health care. This means that we now expect to live to old age, and that most of us are likely to die in hospital surrounded by professional carers and the paraphernalia of medical technology. As recently as the early part of the twentieth century, death was something that usually took place at home, and involved families and neighbours in familiar rituals. The dead person would often be washed and laid out by family members who loved them, and friends and family would gather around the open coffin for a wake, to mourn and bid farewell. The coffin would lie in the family home until the funeral, when it would be carried out of the front door. In many places, the front door was opened only for ceremonial events such as marriages and funerals (the back door being the one for general household use) and people would express their sense of connection to their home by declaring 'I won't leave this place until I am carried out feet first!'.

Nowadays this familiarity with death and dying has been replaced by secrecy, and the business of caring for the dead has been taken over by people who are paid to do it. As Jeffrey Weeks comments, this means that dying has become more fearful for dying people as well as for the bereaved:

Instead of finding ways of coming to terms with the inexorability of our final end we live under its shadow. Death, it often seems, is our dirty or guilty secret, and the victims are those who are dying, often in isolation and terror.[1]

Many writers who deal with the subject of death agree that it is a taboo subject, that mainstream society likes to pretend that death does not exist. They also generally agree that death is a great universal experience, one that we all share. Historically, the downtrodden and oppressed have been comforted by the belief that death, the 'great leveller', was impartial and would take the wealthy and powerful as surely as the poor and weak. This was always an illusion. Except in times of plague and epidemic the rich and powerful have always lived longer and suffered fewer life-threatening illnesses than the poor, a fundamental inequality which persists today. Yet it is understandably tempting to seek for a universal shared experience to bridge painful differences. In an introduction to a collection of their poetry, lesbian writers Suniti Namjoshi and Gillian Hanscombe seem to echo this belief. Everything about lesbian life is different, *except death*:

For us, love is not the same; sex is not the same; parenting is not the same; work is not the same; safety is not the same; respect is not the same; trust is not the same. Only death might, perhaps, be the same.[2]

The question of whether being dead is the same for all human beings is a complex philosophical and spiritual one which cannot be addressed here. However, very little that surrounds death – the experience of dying, the anticipation of death, the processes of grief and bereavement, the feelings of loss, isolation and abandonment, the possible experience of illness and pain, the rituals of funerals and memorial celebrations – is the same for lesbians and non-lesbians. This chapter addresses those things which are special or different about death, dying and bereavement for lesbians, whether the death we are facing is our own or that of a lover, former lover or lesbian friend.

Facing death

Of course, all of us have to come to terms with the knowledge that we must die. For earlier generations this process often had a particular foundation in religious teaching, since most of the world's dominant religions insist that spiritual growth comes from recognition and acceptance of our mortality. It is perhaps too easy to look back on this time with the rose-tinted spectacles of nostalgia: inculcating true believers with the terror that death would come and find them not ready was a profoundly damaging experience for many, and a powerful means of social control. Nevertheless, with the growing secularization of modern life, the acceptance of death as part of life has been replaced by denial, which carries its own psychological, emotional and social costs. 'Because modern life is shaped so much by the exclusion of thoughts of its end, we find it painful and difficult to live with the inevitability of death.'[3] Most of us find it hard to talk about death, and if we do we are often accused of being morbid and depressing. It is easy, therefore, to live as if death was a distant prospect until the (inevitable) moment when events strip us of the comfort of that illusion: because we will die, we try to live as if we are immortal, as if we had an eternity to fulfil our lives' tasks – until death, our own or that of loved ones, finally confronts us.[4]

There is all the difference in the world between the theoretical knowledge that we must all die and the awareness that your own death is likely or imminent. Because our societies fear and deny death there is general agreement that it is better for a dying person *not* to know that they are dying. Sometimes this may be true. It is always traumatic to be told that you are dying, and some people want to be protected from that knowledge, drawing on the comfort of denial until the last. However, a dying person is all too often kept in ignorance in an effort to protect those around them, who would find it too difficult to handle the situation otherwise. Sometimes a dying person, or those close to them, will know or suspect that they are dying, despite the reassuring lies of those around them. One elderly lesbian mourning the death of her life partner of almost fifty years told me, 'They sent her home from the hospital and told me it wasn't cancer and she would get better. But I saw it on her notes, carcinoma. They could at least have told me the truth. What was it, did they think I was too stupid to know?'

If you have been told that you are dying, you will probably experience many conflicting emotions as you pass through the stages of grief. As a lesbian, the difficult task of coming to terms with dying may be both complicated and enriched by your lesbianism. You may feel great fear, loneliness, grief, anger, or despair, perhaps mixed up with feelings which are difficult to accept or understand. You may feel furious at people who will be alive after you have gone, guilty at the pain you will be causing by your death, frustrated at the list of things you always meant to do and now cannot, vengeful at those who have done you wrong in the past. There may be delightful positive feelings which disconcert, surprise or comfort you. You may feel a sense of relief or euphoria at surrendering responsibility and giving up the hard struggle to keep going. You may feel liberated from daily concerns, curious about the experience of dying or filled to overflowing with love and tenderness for people and things that have been dear to you. Sometimes your feelings may frighten you with their intensity, or may seem irrational or unacceptable. You may experience strong feelings about your family of origin: a longing for the closeness or acceptance which you never had from them, a desire to settle unfinished business, gratitude and joy in their closeness and support, or grief that perhaps you are to die before one or both of your parents.

If you are religious, belief may be enormously helpful, or may seem to fail you just when you most need it. On the other hand, beliefs which you have chosen to leave behind with the other things of childhood may return unexpectedly. It can be extremely difficult to make sense of the spiritual aspect of your death. You may need to move through new ways of thinking about the world, ways which may be alien to those around you who are accustomed to a familiar you and are uncomfortable with you seeming to move on to different spiritual ground. This can be especially difficult for lesbians, since organized patriarchal religion is so hostile to our existence that many (if not most) lesbians straightforwardly reject anything that smacks of spirituality. On the other hand, some lesbian communities have developed alternative woman-centred spiritual traditions and rituals, and, if these have been an important part of your life, they can offer great comfort in the face of death.

As a lesbian, any or all of these emotional challenges may be made more difficult, or easier, or simply different, by your sexuality. If religious and spiritual questions are or become central for you at this time, you may find yourself troubled by the unforgiving anti-lesbian doctrines of your religious heritage. You may find yourself plunged all over again into struggles that you thought you had dealt with long ago. If your religion has taught you that lesbian love is sinful, or that you will spend eternity in hell for following your desires, such teachings may take on a new and disturbing power in the face of death. Lesbians who have had a religious upbringing have all had to find ways of surviving these cruel teachings, and those who have not may have no way of understanding how powerful such beliefs can be when we are vulnerable. It may be very hard, if you have a partner who is unconcernedly agnostic, for her to support you through these painful questions, and many of your lesbian friends may be unwilling even to pay attention to them. It may be helpful for you to remember that hatred of lesbians is found *not* in the holy texts of the great religions but in the interpretations of religious institutions. It is frightened men who have taught that lesbian love is sinful, not any god. If you were brought up in a Jewish or Christian tradition, you may find comfort in the work of lesbian and gay theologians who make a clear distinction between the word of God and the prejudices of human beings in the religious hierarchy (see Further Reading), or from a lesbian or gay priest or rabbi.

One of the most painful things about confronting death is the loneliness. You may be surrounded by people who love and care for you deeply, but you are about to leave them, and nothing can alter that. However much you love them and they you, you must let go. Again, being a lesbian may add to the complexities of this letting go. If your parents do not accept your lesbianism, or are hostile to your lover and friends, you may fear that they will somehow exploit the accepted status of their relationship to you (in contrast to the generally unaccepted and invisible status of your relationship with lovers and friends) in order to muscle in as you become less able to put up a fight. You may fear that those whom you dearly want to be with you as you die will be excluded. This fear can be at least partly assuaged. Much depends on your place of death. If you wish and are able to die in your own home, it is relatively easy to retain control over who spends time with you. It is important that you make absolutely clear, to as many people as possible, who you do and do not want to visit you, so that your wishes may be carried out if it becomes difficult for you to communicate. If you anticipate dying in a hospital or hospice, you should be able to have your wishes met there too. One positive consequence of the HIV/AIDS pandemic is that many hospitals and hospices are more aware and respectful of lesbian and gay relationships and community ties than they have traditionally been, and if you are able to talk openly with your health care team, you should be able to ensure that they know and respect your wishes about who should be treated as next of kin. If you anticipate the possibility that you may be taken to a hospital or hospice which is new to you, it may be helpful to make a living will setting out your wishes. The legal status of such documents varies from place to place, but most medical and nursing staff prefer to respect the documented wishes of their dying patients. If you have reason to anticipate hostility and trouble of a major sort – perhaps you suspect that your parents or grandparents will try to take your kids away from the care of your partner, or will make strenuous efforts to get an unwanted religious ritual carried out over your deathbed – you may wish to get lesbian-friendly legal advice about the various ways in which you can legally restrain those individuals from harassing you.

The prospect of leaving behind those we love most deeply is extremely painful, and may give rise to the belief that we will in some way fail or betray them by our death, or to fears about how they will manage on their own. Again, being a lesbian can add a special dimension to this. If you have a partner you may feel guilty at the pain your death will cause her, pain which can only be harder to bear in a society that refuses to recognize the love which can exist between two women. As women we are brought up to take care of other people, and it can be very hard to stop doing this, even when we are dying. You may be anguished at your inability to continue caring for the woman you love after your death. On the other hand, you may be shocked and distressed at feelings of resentment towards her when you imagine her eventually forgetting you and starting a new relationship with another woman. You may be tormented by fantasies of her in the arms of some woman you heartily dislike, or even by the suspicion that she will 'go straight' and fall in love with a man.

It helps to recognize that these feelings are a natural product of your powerlessness to control the future, and that they may also point to things in your relationship which you feel insecure or vulnerable about. It will be hard for both of you to resist the temptation to fantasize about a future in which you will still be 'together' in some way. Such fantasies can be very comforting, but beware of attaching too much emotional force to them. They soon cease to be a comfort if you are struggling with guilt because you got her to promise she wouldn't look at another woman again, or if she is struggling with guilt because she has felt pressured into making promises to you that she knows she cannot keep. Be gentle with yourself and with each other; your lives have been spent in the constant battering of homophobia and it is understandable if that has left a legacy of confusing feelings as you approach death.

Another worry may be how difficult the world can make it for the surviving member of a lesbian couple. Diane Silver, who survived her partner of seven years, describes how cruelly and offensively the heterosexual world treated her as she dealt with the practicalities of her lover's death:

An insurance company . . . suggested that I was a con artist who took care of Patty to gain control of her property. The obituary writer objected to listing me first among the survivors – that placement was reserved for spouses. Besides, the writer argued, how could he be sure that Patty and I really were 'companions'. When I had to get certified copies of Patty's death certificate to file her income taxes, the clerk . . . asked: 'Can you prove your relationship?'[5]

Dealing with all the practicalities which follow a death is difficult enough, without having to deal with anti-lesbian hostility from the heterosexual establishment. But this is one time when knowing that your death is imminent is a gift. While you are still well enough, you can sort out many of the practicalities yourself, or can get legal advice on appointing an executor or someone with power of attorney to shoulder the burden after your death. If you have a partner, discuss this carefully with her. Many lovers want to sort out the business aspect of their partner's death for themselves, but it may in fact be a much better idea for a trusted friend to take this on. However expected a death is, it will almost certainly still come as a great emotional shock, and although keeping busy and being very practical can seem like a good idea, it is not always possible to predict how painful and difficult it will prove to be in reality. If you do decide to ask a friend, discuss things with them in as much detail as possible, and involve your lover in these discussions as much (or as little) as she wants to be involved. This is the best way in which you can care for the needs of both yourself and your partner.

One place where you may be able to get lesbian-friendly advice and information about all the practicalities of dealing with death is your local AIDS organization or gay bereavement group (see local gay press, or the phone book). AIDS has brought death and dying to

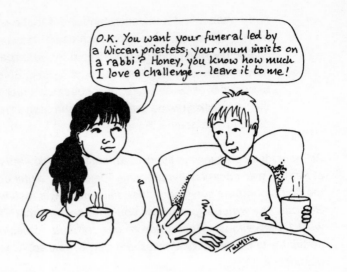

the forefront for many thousands of gay men, and this is the community which knows most about living wills, gay-friendly funeral directors and other important issues.

A good death?

It is generally those who are terminally ill who know roughly when they are likely to die and who have time to prepare. Those who die as a direct result of serious injury usually live for a relatively short time after their injury, and are likely to be unconscious or confused during that time. So, if you know the likely time of your death, you will be facing the realities of your illness. These are likely to include pain, growing incapacity and perhaps confusion. We fear all of these, and trying to plan for a 'good death' means making arrangements in advance so that you know these possibilities are taken care of. Discuss pain relief options well in advance with your health adviser. If possible, do some research into pain relief for yourself, or ask someone to do so for you. No doctor or alternative practitioner can be expected to know all there is to know about pain relief, and there are many ways of tackling pain. You may chose the certainty of drugs – properly administered these need not cause confusion – in which case, try to see a pain specialist to discuss which kind of drug treatment is best for your condition. There are now specialist pain clinics, whose expertise in the subject is growing rapidly, and you may be able to access this kind of care. Alternatively, specialist cancer nurses and hospice care staff are very well informed about pain treatment. In Britain, if you have cancer, you can ask to see a specialist nurse from one of the cancer charities, in particular the Macmillan Trust, who will visit you at home. This can make an enormous difference, since the Macmillan nurses have a wealth of specialist knowledge about the physical and emotional needs of a dying person and those close to her.

If you distrust drugs, alternative pain relief strategies such as visualization, acupuncture or herbalism can be extremely effective, and it is increasingly likely that these will be available to you in a hospital or hospice setting. If you have a real fear of drugs such as morphine (still the analgesic of choice for much terminal care), it is worth discussing their use with your doctor and getting as much information as you can. Although large doses of morphine can cause you to feel 'doped up', and may give rise to distressingly vivid dreams or hallucinations, alternative analgesics and up-to-date techniques for delivering morphine mean that such distressing experiences should now be uncommon. Given the risks of living as a lesbian, it is understandable that we want to stay in control as much as possible, and choosing pain relief that will enable you to do that can be very empowering.

Issues such as pain relief, basic nursing care, privacy and the degree of control you are able to take during your last few days determine whether you want to die in a hospital, a hospice or at home. Most pain relief should now be available to those who choose to die at home, although the bulk of nursing care will almost certainly have to be provided by friends and family members. Most GP practices in Britain have community nurses whose responsibilities include providing care for dying patients, but there are many demands on their time. On the other hand, hospitals are very hectic and busy places and, however hard their staff try to ensure continuity of care for terminally ill patients, this is not always possible. You may fear the homophobia of nursing staff in a hospital. Much hard work is being done in some hospitals to ensure that lesbian and gay patients are treated with respect, but this is not the case everywhere. However, there is growing awareness in the nursing profession that good terminal care is holistic care, and you should find that your sexuality and relationships are respected.

The hospice movement was started to give people the chance to die as well and as peacefully as possible. Hospices recognize the spiritual aspect of death and dying, but are unlikely to force it on to you. They are probably more likely than most hospitals to have an accepting attitude to lesbian and gay people, and they have expertise in pain relief and the nursing needs of people who are dying. Most of them are run by charities, and although they do not charge for their services they will be very grateful for any donation or bequest which you are able to make. The downside is that there may not be a hospice near you. It is also important to remember that hospices are there specifically for dying people. They generally take people for the last few days of their life, so you will have to make other arrangements up until that point. You may also have to plan as far ahead as possible to ensure that there will be space for you.

Given the choice, most of us would probably elect to die at home, in our own beds, surrounded by our own things and by those closest to us. For lesbians this may be still more important, since we may have become accustomed to thinking of our home as a sanctuary from the outside world. With modern pain relief techniques there is no reason why dying at home should not be as comfortable as in a hospital, and there are many other advantages. You will not have to stick to hospital routines, to worry about confronting staff or other patients who are uninformed about or hostile towards lesbians, to worry about whether your decisions about visitors or treatment will be respected or to leave your children, pets, plants or garden. However, there are some aspects of dying at home which may need careful thought and preparation. If you are housebound or confined to bed, you may well feel at times as if your house has become your prison. If your partner is providing the bulk of your care, she may need somewhere to escape to once in a while to recuperate and recharge her batteries. And it can be hard to relinquish control of the day-to-day running of your house, to see it become filled with the paraphernalia of sickness or to lose it bit by bit as you become less able to move around in it. As we die, our horizons gradually diminish. You may begin by changing from full-time to part-time work, then by stopping work, then moving around a smaller area of your neighbourhood, then never moving beyond the garden, then never leaving the house, then by being unable to climb the stairs, by becoming confined to one room, eventually spending your final days or hours in a little bubble of space gradually shrinking around your bed. This process is in some ways a kind of reversal of what happened as we grew up, and you may experience it as terrifying and frustrating or comforting and reassuring.

Whether it is a positive or negative experience partly depends on how pleasant it is to spend time in the place where your bed is located and on how reconciled you are able to be to your death. It is therefore well worth spending time while you are able on deciding which part of your home you feel most at ease in. It may be possible to hire or borrow a hospital-style bed on locking castors; if your house is large enough, this bed may be moved from one room to another, or even out into the garden. Many of the tasks of nursing you will be easier on such a bed, so it is worth seeing if one is available for you. You may wish to prepare for a possibly lengthy period of time in one small space by making sure that it is made easy for you to listen to your favourite music, that you can control the heat and light in the room yourself, that you are able to open and close the curtains or blinds yourself, that you can call someone to you without exerting yourself too much (perhaps by ringing a bell or blowing a whistle), and that it is easy and pleasant for family, friends, children and pets to come into and out of your room and to spend time in it. If you don't have a television or video recorder, consider renting them or borrowing one from a friend: some people find television a good way of staying in touch with the outside world, and you may appreciate this when your other activities are so restricted. Make sure televisions and videos have a remote control so that you can control them from your bed when needed. Get a telephone by your bed, and make sure that it has a ring that can be switched off for times when you need to sleep. If you love reading but cannot hold a book, there are special tables and clamps designed for this purpose – ask at your local hospital or GP surgery. If you would love to be read to, suggest to your friends that they set up a reading rota. Dogs may need to be exercised, and again it is helpful if friends can share in this, so that your partner does not have to do it all. With foresight and careful planning, these last days at home can be sweet and comforting for everyone involved.

Bereavement: loss and grief

Bereavement can happen at any time in our lives, and at any stage in a relationship. There is a generally shared recognition of how hard it is to lose a parent or spouse, but since lesbian relationships are rarely honoured in mainstream society our losses are seldom recognized. Grieiving for the death of a lover is one of the hardest things anyone has to face, and it is too often made harder and more bitter by those who deny or belittle our love. In many ways an expected death offers opportunities that are denied to those bereaved suddenly and unexpectedly – opportunities to say some of the important things we leave unsaid and to tie up loose ends – but, however much you believe you have come to terms with a long-anticipated death, the first reaction is usually shock.

The emotional process of grief is sometimes said to pass through clear steps or stages, but in fact things are seldom so clear-cut and it is probably more helpful to think in terms of the *elements* of grieving. The recognized elements of grief following loss include shock, numbness, disbelief or denial, anger, depression or despair and – yes, it comes eventually – acceptance. These elements are often present in other traumatic losses such as the ending of a relationship or the loss of a job or home, but they are most overwhelming following a bereavement. People who have been bereaved report disturbing experiences such as suddenly recognizing the dead person in the street or a crowd, hearing their voice, being woken by dreams or nightmares in which they are vividly present or simply forgetting that they have died. Such experiences may take on added stress if your relationship has been kept secret from friends or work colleagues since, if this is the case, you may feel the need to hide the extremes of your grief. Whether or not you face this added burden, the intensity and vividness of these 'hauntings' can make you feel frightened and vulnerable. It helps to know that they are very common experiences shared by many bereaved people, and it is especially important at this time for you to get whatever support you can. Lesbian theologian Elizabeth Stuart recognizes that the comfort of others during bereavement is particularly important to lesbians and gay men: 'When a gay or lesbian person dies', she writes, 'a great deal of additional pain can result . . . partner and friends may even be excluded from the services, with the result that the funeral becomes a farce, a lie.'[6]

The physical stresses of grief are not always recognized, but it is important to understand that grief is exhausting physically as well as emotionally, and you should be as gentle as possible with yourself at this time. It may be tempting to bury yourself in work or to throw your energies into taking charge of all the practicalities which follow on the heels of a death, but try to resist doing this. Rest as much as possible. You are likely to find sleep very difficult at first, or very unpredictable, but resting as deeply as possible is almost as good as sleeping, and will help minimize the effects of broken sleep. Try to lie down in a warm and comfortable spot, close your eyes and let your body relax as much as possible. This can feel scary; many of us feel that the strength of our grief threatens to overwhelm us, and we resist being quiet and unoccupied in order not to allow our feelings to well up. The truth is that, painful and terrible although it may feel, your grief is a good and loving gift to the woman you have lost, and is the path to healing for yourself. Powerful though these feelings are, they will not overwhelm you. You may feel as if your loss and misery will drag you down past the point of no return, but life is not so easily quenched and you *will* bob up again at the right time. Allow yourself as much time to cry and rage as you can. You may find it impossible to cry in front of anyone else, or too scary to do it on your own. Trust these feelings and try to get what you need. It is of course best to grieve with other lesbians or close friends who knew and loved the woman who has died but, if you are very isolated and cannot easily do this, get in touch with a bereavement support group or with your local lesbian line or lesbian and gay switchboard. Heterosexual bereavement support groups (such as CRUSE) can be very helpful: grief is such a profound experience that it tends to override mundane prejudices. When Diane Silver's lover died, she found this support contrasted markedly with the hostility of the heterosexual mainstream:

Since Patty died, one group of heterosexuals has not questioned my right to call myself a widow. In fact, they were the first people to give me that label. Their emmissary was a woman who called me a few weeks after Patty died. 'Did you know that I was also widowed young?' my acquaintance asked. 'Let's talk.'[7]

It is not only emotional support that you will need. Practical tasks such as shopping, cleaning, walking the dogs or doing laundry may feel beyond you for a while. Do not be ashamed to ask for help with these tasks. Nor should you be frightened by the sometimes unexpected physical effects of grief. If you have not passed the menopause, these may include upsets to your menstrual cycle – you may stop bleeding altogether, your periods may become irregular for a time or you may find that you bleed very heavily. You may feel nauseous or dizzy, may lose your appetite or feel ravenously hungry, and may experience aches and pains in unexpected places. Some women describe feelings of emptiness or hollowness inside.

One inevitable consequence of the death of your lover is that you lose your sexual partner. Bereavement can cause strange or upsetting changes in our sexuality, and these changes can take on additional significance for lesbians, since our sexuality is in any case so widely censured. You may feel sexually dead, and as if you can never imagine being sexual with anyone again. On the other hand, you may be surprised or disturbed by powerful sexual feelings, or by erotic dreams or fantasies about your dead lover. It can be devastating to wake from an intimate dream in which you were sharing sexual pleasure with a beloved woman to find yourself in an empty bed and remember that she is dead. These deep sexual feelings can come up whatever happened between you while she was still alive. She may have died unexpectedly at the beginning of a new love affair, or you may have spent years together and settled into comfortable intimacy with lots of cuddles and less frequent sex. If she died after a long illness, you may have thought that you had let go of the sexual contact between you. Whatever happened while she was alive, try to accept that your body needs to find its own path towards letting go of your sexual connection with her.

If you still have feelings of guilt or unease about being a lesbian (and it is a rare lesbian who doesn't), these feelings may disgust or horrify you. It may feel deeply inappropriate or even disrespectful to have sexual feelings about someone who is dead. In fact, the reverse is true. Such feelings reflect the reality of the sexual link between you. Try to honour them and make them part of your grieving. If you have fantasies about your dead lover which arouse you, there is nothing shameful or inappropriate about masturbating and remembering the pleasure you used to enjoy with her, even if that was a long time in the past. This can be a very deep and intimate way of celebrating the love that you shared, and of soothing your grieving body with loving touch, as she might have done.

On the other hand, you may find yourself attracted to other women, fantasizing or dreaming about sex with other women (or men), or simply feeling sexual in a highly charged but undirected way. This does not mean that you are being disloyal to your dead partner, simply that this is how you feel right now. It should go without saying that you do not have to act on these feelings. Getting involved in messy situations is not what you need when you are recovering from your lover's death, and starting a new relationship before you are ready to move on from the loss of your partner will not be fair on you or the new girlfriend. But one of the joys of being a lesbian is that casual sexual encounters carry far less potential risk than the heterosexual equivalent, and, if sex with no strings attached is a familiar and reassuring part of your life, there is no reason why you should not fall back on it now. Don't forget that you are especially vulnerable, and that strong feelings may be sparked off by having sex. It is only fair to warn potential sex partners if you are likely to become upset, and you do need to take care of yourself as well. Casual sex can be a much-needed distraction from the miseries of grieving, but this in itself can get in the way of coming to terms with your loss and eventually moving forward. A good rule of thumb is, if you find yourself doing something which you know you will never be able to tell your best friend, it is probably something which you will regret.

Grief often feels intolerable and it can be very tempting to obliterate it or deaden it with alcohol, drugs, sex or busy-ness. It may help to recognize that you *are* struggling to deal with something very hard: losing a lover or child is probably the hardest thing for any human being to cope with. And it is also important to hold in your mind the knowledge that you will not feel like this for ever. One of the most painful things about great grief is that it shuts you away from the world, and it can feel as if this is what life is going to be like from now on. But this is not true. Grief is a journey, a process, and it changes all the time. Little by little, things will shift and happiness will become possible again.

In the desolate hour, there is an outcry; a clenching of the hands upon emptiness; a burning pain of bereavement; a weary ache of loss. But anguish, like ecstasy, is not forever. There comes a gentleness, a returning quietness, a restoring stillness. This, too, is a door to life.[8]

Alcohol, drugs, binge-eating or compulsive busy-ness can all deaden the pain, but in the long run they do not help, because they get in the way of the natural process of grieving. On the other hand, some lesbians can be a little insensitive about how hard it is to manage bereavement. Don't feel that you have to be the 'perfect' mourner and get it absolutely 'right', or that you have done something dreadful if you get drunk a couple of times. But do trust that your grief *is* bearable (it is *your* grief, after all) and that it will resolve itself in a way that is right for you.

Funerals and all that business

In order to make this journey through grief, we need our rituals of mourning. This can be an extremely painful time for lesbian and gay mourners, as we are all too often shut out of the ceremonies of biological families and religious institutions. By excluding us from funerals, wakes, sitting shiva or other mourning rituals, people whose relationship to the dead woman was socially recognized are able to deny the reality of her lesbianism. This exclusion robs us of the recognition which our love and grief demand, and can turn the healing process of mourning into a bitter, angry and lonely struggle.

It is important, if this happens, that we work with friends to create our own ceremonies and rituals of grieving. As Elizabeth Stuart writes, 'It is extremely important to come together as friends, for in grief we need others, particularly if our right to grieve is being denied.'[9] The enormity of your loss may make you feel that no ceremony could ever be enough, that rituals such as lighting candles or meeting to share memories of the woman you have lost are silly and pointless. But do not underestimate the power of such small acts in helping you to unlock your grief, share your loss and get loving support at this time when you most need it:

whatever ceremony is chosen – big or small, public or private, conventional or innovative – it can be a kind of punctuation mark, an ending and a beginning, a way to help the survivor to move on to the next emotional step.[10]

The kinds of funerals and mourning rituals chosen are important. It may be that the woman whose death you are mourning and whose life you are celebrating was able to plan her funeral and/or memorial gathering beforehand. If so, there will be great comfort in knowing that what will happen is what she wanted. Even if this was not possible, you will be able to draw on your intimate knowledge of her to make sure this important ritual is what she would have chosen if she could have done. Things which can be helpful at such ceremonies are:

- playing a piece of music which she particularly loved, or which evokes the kind of person she was

- reading a poem, or the words of a song, which was important to her, or to both of you, or which express something of what you are feeling

- asking people who knew and loved her to speak for a few minutes about what she meant to them

- asking people to bring a small gift for her; something which would have pleased her when she was alive. You can collect these together and either burn them on a small bonfire or bury them in your garden or a favourite place of hers.

Such small rituals can be especially important when we are refused access to the burial or cremation, but may also be shared between close friends in addition to a more public ceremony. If you are able to, you may wish to say a special goodbye by scattering her ashes, either alone or with a small group of friends. If you are unable to do this, you could burn something personal, such as a piece of her clothing or a photograph, and scatter that instead. You may want to acknowledge and celebrate her life as a lesbian, and this can be done in many ways. You may choose to enclose favourite lesbian books in her coffin, or to bury her wearing the lesbian symbols which were important to her in life (such as a labyris earring or her freedom rings), or to collect for a memorial which celebrates your relationship or includes some other reference to her lesbianism. Alternative spiritual rituals based on goddess worship or other feminist woman-centred practices and symbols may be an important part of this for you. Small gestures of defiant celebration such as this can be especially healing if others are denying or attempting to hide this truth about her life.

Of course, people have very different needs at a time like this. For example, many mourners gain great comfort from reading Henry Scott-Holland's elegaic paragraph on death, which starts 'Death is nothing at all. I have only slipped away into the next room.' Yet, in a piece on grieving the loss of so many gay men with AIDS, Simon Watney writes, 'I think this is an appalling prayer. I think it makes mourning impossible.'[11] Of course, the words which make mourning 'impossible' for one person may be the most important source of comfort to another. At this time above all else, you must do what feels right.

Losing someone to suicide: a special grief

It is now recognized that losing someone through suicide has an enormous impact on the grieving process. One of the most devastating consequences of heterosexism is that the suicide rates for lesbians are higher than they are for non-lesbian women. Lesbians are more likely to have the experience of surviving a lover or close friend who killed herself, although this is not recognized in the self-help books addressed to survivors of suicide.

For lesbians mourning someone who has taken her own life, there is a complex double burden of grief and stigma. All survivors of suicide have to deal with the impulse (or social and familial pressure) to hide or deny the fact that suicide was the cause of death. All survivors of suicide face an appalling sense of abandonment; this person has chosen to leave you in the most final and irrevocable way possible, with no argument, and in doing so has left you to deal with the consequences for yourself and by yourself. The death of a loved person, however much it was anticipated, inevitably gives rise to feelings of anger at being abandoned. When the death was deliberately self-inflicted, these feelings of anger can become the most central part of your emotional reaction to your loss. Of course it is confusing and difficult to feel anger against someone who is dead. This is especially true when they were unhappy enough to kill themselves: it seems that the 'right' response is pity and sorrow rather than anger. So the experience of anger may leave us deeply ashamed, guilty or horrified. We may refuse to recognize our anger, deny it, bury it or turn it against ourselves or some scapegoat whom we seek to blame for the suicide. Scapegoating is a particularly common response: a little bit of scapegoating seems to be practiced even by people who are dealing quite well with survivorship. It helps them with the intensity of the anger welling up inside.[12]

Unfortunately, this may mean that others – parents in particular – may scapegoat the dead woman's lesbianism as the 'cause' of her suicide. They may blame you, as her lover or friend, and may even accuse her lesbian friends or partners of having 'made her' a lesbian and dragged her into this unhappy life. Because lesbianism is stigmatized, such accusations may remain unpleasantly buried, as this account shows. Here, the surviving boyfriend and mother of a young woman who killed herself make a scapegoat of her female friend at college:

It was a very tumultuous friendship with a woman that she had . . . If they hadn't met, if she hadn't gone to that college, she might still be alive. It was a very strange, tortured relationship, the nature of which we still don't understand. But Beth's first attempt [at suicide] had directly to do with her friend's behaviour in rejecting her.[13]

The heterosexism of most writers on suicide means that accounts such as this remain buried and that the scapegoating of lesbian survivors of suicide remains invisible. So, too, does the grief of lesbians who have lost lovers and friends through suicide. Yet it helps to recognize that the impulse to deflect anger by scapegoating others is common to all survivors of suicide, and that, if you are searching for someone to blame or if you are scapegoated yourself, this is not happening 'just' because you are a lesbian.

If your lover has killed herself, you will be facing a particularly difficult and traumatic grieving process. All survivors of suicide are tormented by the feeling that they could not have loved the dead person enough, or they could have prevented them killing themselves. This may be additionally agonising for lesbians. Since lesbian love is seldom taken seriously, and since your lover chose to die rather than stay in her relationship with you, you may start to question not only whether you loved her enough but whether lesbian love can ever be 'real', or can ever be enough, or whether indeed you have the right to call yourself her lover at all. You may feel that your love for her, your relationship to her, or even your lesbian identity, are unimportant or unreal. Again, remind yourself that the feeling of failure and inadequacy is common to all who survive suicide, and that you would probably be having similar feelings even if you were not a lesbian.

Because suicide is always traumatic – there is never time to say goodbye or to prepare for death – and because so many extra burdens of guilt, anger, shame and fear are associated with mourning someone who has killed herself, it is even more important to get help and support. It is also especially important to have adequate rituals and opportunities to celebrate the life of the person you have lost. There seems to be a general feeling that a death by suicide is best hushed up, and all too often the normal rituals of mourning are set aside:

Funerals or memorial services help many people define how they feel about the dead person. But . . . many survivors [of suicide] avoid any formal marking of the death. By not holding a memorial service or even a funeral, they deprive themselves of an early opportunity to mourn and to mark what was valuable in the life that has been lost.[14]

Even if your feelings of loss, despair, anger and abandonment feel overwhelming, *do* take the time to carry out those rituals of grieving which you know your lost lover or friend would have wanted. Then try to recognize that you are entitled to have help in healing from this. More than any other kind of death, suicide leaves a permament mark on your life. You will not forget. But you *will* move on, and your feelings will find their proper place in your future life, if you are able to go through the difficult and sometimes unpredictable task of grieving. The best and most important help you can get is talking. Talk, in any circumstances you can and to whoever is appropriate and available, about every aspect of this death and its effects on your life. Get professional help from a therapist, counsellor or specialist bereavement group. Ring your local gay bereavement project or lesbian and gay counselling project, talk to friends and colleagues, ring the Samaritains.

Don't set yourself to mourn as if it is a project to be completed before a certain time. Grief has its own timetable and its own schedule, and your best approach is to trust that the healing processes within you will demand what is needed and take whatever time is required. Life *is* still there ahead of you and, however despairing you feel right now, it *does* hold new possibilities of love and happiness. This, too, will pass.

Endword:
the consequences of AIDS

The impact of HIV disease on gay communities has been immense, and gay men living in many areas are confronted with the need to deal with an overwhelming number of deaths. This has an impact on lesbians too. We too are losing friends and loved ones to HIV, both lesbians and our gay men friends, as well as bisexual and heterosexual friends and/or lovers. The impact of the epidemic has meant that lesbian and gay communities are learning new ways of responding to death, and that may mean that lesbians who are bereaved or who are facing their own death can find better support than they might otherwise have done. However, if we are not careful, the sheer scale of the HIV pandemic can make us unable to take our own losses seriously. Certainly, this has not been helped by some thoughtless gay activists who have responded angrily to lesbians voicing concern about HIV or about other diseases which are more significant to lesbians. We have been accused of 'virus envy', and gay men have not shown as much willingness to campaign for lesbian health issues as lesbians have to campaign around HIV/AIDS. If you live in one of the epicentres of HIV, the idea of dealing with one lesbian dying may seem somehow less important than the experience of gay men who may have lost dozens of friends and lovers. But one death is *enough* to deal with. It is precisely because large numbers of deaths are too much to deal with that gay communities are carrying such an emotional and psychological burden at present. If you have cause to grieve for one person (whether yourself, a friend or a lover), that is your need and your right. Allowing your own grief to be diminished by the 'larger' griefs of others makes about as much sense as refusing to enjoy lesbian sex because millions of heterosexual women can't enjoy it too. Death and dying have important differences for lesbians, and our communities are evolving ways of recognizing and dealing with that fact. But it is still very early days, and you are doing something very difficult. Take it easy.

Further reading

There is a dearth of material available for lesbians dealing with death and dying. Pick up any lesbian anthology at random and try to find the section on death! However, although this list has few lesbian-specific books, all the ones listed here are useful and helpful.

For or about lesbians

Audre Lorde, *The Cancer Journals* (London: Sheba, 1980). Very moving and inspiring diary of Lorde's struggle with breast cancer.

Elizabeth Stuart, *Daring to Speak Love's Name: a Gay and Lesbian Prayer Book* (London: Hamish Hamilton, 1992). Contains useful suggestions for funeral and memorial rituals, not all of which are Christian, together with some useful contact addresses.

Daniel Helminiak, *What the Bible Really Says about Homosexuality* (San Francisco: Alamo Square Press, 1994). Very useful for those seeking a lesbian-affirmative Christianity.

For or about women

Rosa Ainley, *Death of a Mother: Daughters' Stories* (London: Pandora, 1991).

Sarah Boston, *Too Deep for Tears: Eighteen Years after the Death of My Son, Will* (London: Pandora, 1993).

Jean Shapiro (US edition Paula Brown Doress and Diana Laskin Siegal), *Ourselves, Growing Older: Women Ageing with Knowledge and Power*

(London: Fontana, 1989). Good section on preparing for death, with useful contact listings.

Sheila Kitzinger, *Woman's Experience of Sex* (London: Dorling Kindersley, 1983). Has a section on bereavement.

Surviving suicide

Alison Werthheimer, *A Special Scar: The Experiences of People Bereaved by Suicide* (London: Routledge, 1991).

Christopher Lukas and Henry M. Seiden, *Silent Grief: Living in the Wake of Suicide* (London: Macmillan, 1987).

In the United States, the American Association of Suicidology publishes *The Care of the Suicide Survivor*, in association with some survivors' groups.

Practicalities

The Consumer's Association publishes a booklet, *What to Do When Someone Dies*: write to them at 14 Buckingham Street, London WC2.

9 Are You Being Served? Getting the Best Care Possible

The women's health movement has had very real benefits in terms of improving the standard of health care which women receive,[1] and there is an ongoing activist struggle to achieve high-quality health and social care by women's groups, black and minority ethnic groups, disability rights groups, elders' rights groups and gay rights groups. Lesbians are, of course, found in all these groups, but we are more than likely to be marginalized, tokenized or silenced altogether within them.[2] The experience of lesbians who have had to fight for their place in their own communities of origin may be particularly draining, especially in the face of serious or chronic illness, as Audre Lorde's passionate words signal:

We all have to die at least once. Making that death useful would be winning for me. I wasn't supposed to exist anyway, not in any meaningful way in this fucked-up whiteboys' world. I want desperately to live, and I'm ready to fight for that living, even if I die shortly.[3]

The complex multiple oppressions experienced by most lesbians have not been faced in silence. Just as black women have organized around their own health in response to their marginalization in the women's health movement, many thousands of lesbians are networking, organizing and agitating to get lesbian issues on to the health agenda. This activism has increased in a dramatic and exciting way in the last few years. This is no doubt related to the enormous swell of gay political activism around the HIV pandemic, and to our recognition that concern about HIV was threatening to drown out the few voices speaking about health issues of more direct concern to lesbians. It is also no doubt connected to the very visible successes of the feminist health movement – now active on every continent – and to the very real changes in social perceptions of homosexuality[4] which have made it more possible for lesbian health and social care professionals to be out in the context of their work and to be promoting lesbian issues.

Whatever the historical reasons behind it, lesbian health is slowly but surely creeping on to the agenda. Nevertheless, the reality is that homophobia and heterosexism remain profoundly entrenched. The medical profession has been instrumental in creating and justifying homophobia, and homophobic attitudes, beliefs and practices remain the norm among health and social care practitioners. There is no excuse or justification for homophobic care, but, if lesbians want to receive the high-quality services which are our right, we still have to be prepared to confront issues that non-lesbian women don't have to deal with. This chapter outlines the current state of play for lesbians using health care services (whether private, state-run or voluntary) and suggests some strategies for getting our needs recognized and met.

Change needed: an overview of problems with services

Whatever health care infrastructure exists in your locality – whether you have state-run health care free at the point of need (as in Britain or Scandinavian countries), a largely private service run for profit and requiring you to have your own insurance policy (as in the USA) or a mix of public and private (as in Germany) – the service is highly unlikely to recognize that lesbian clients exist. For example, in one survey of gynaecologists in the USA, *half* claimed never to have seen a lesbian patient,[5] while one British consultant was so ignorant of lesbianism that he believed we all have enlarged clitorises and abnormal body hair.[6]

❝ I told the nurse examining me that I am a lesbian, because I thought it might be relevant. She didn't say anything at first, and then she looked at me and asked 'Well, have you ever had sex?' What she meant was had I ever had real sex, i.e., sex with a man! ❞

'Janet'

Health and social care professionals have an absolute obligation to provide the best care possible to all their clients with no exception. The appalling record of ignorance about lesbian health and the mistreatment which lesbians have experienced are inexcusable. There is now a copious amount of research into lesbians' interactions with the health care profession in the USA, Canada, Australia, Britain and mainland Europe, and several key themes have emerged.

- Lesbianism is understood by many people working in health and social care to be either a pathology in its own right or a direct cause of pathology. This is especially true in the field of mental health.[7]

- There is general and widespread ignorance about lesbians, lesbianism and the health concerns of lesbians.[8]

- There is discrimination against lesbians working as doctors and nurses or in the professions allied to medicine. This means that we are less likely to have access to lesbian health care workers, and that the homophobia and heterosexism of the profession remains hard to challenge.[9]

- Lesbians and our partners and lesbian friends often receive discriminatory or offensive treatment from medical and nursing staff when in hospital.[10] This may extend to a refusal to recognize partners as next of kin, an issue which may be devastating for lesbians in intensive care units or who are terminally ill.

- We may face direct hostility and open expressions of bigotry from those who are supposed to be providing our care. Research into the attitudes of nursing staff to lesbians repeatedly uncovers extremely negative attitudes. Not untypical is the nurse who wrote that 'They are sick. They are not normal human beings. They try to turn young, normal people into lesbians with their gay marches.'[11]

- Even those health care workers who are aware of homophobia and reject it may present problems for lesbian clients. Lesbians may be 'subjected to monologues, lectures and anecdotes designed to convince them that the practitioner is not sexist, heterosexist or homophobic'.[12]

- All too often, lesbians are put into a position where they are expected to educate and inform health care professionals about lesbian issues. This may range from embarrassed questioning on the part of curious nurses, to detailed interrogation from medical staff, to having to be proactive and well-informed about lesbian health issues which doctors may know relatively little about.[13] Some lesbians in one survey 'reported that they spent an exorbitant amount of their health care time educating providers about lesbianism and dissuading them from sterotypes'.[14]

> This is a daunting list, and of course it comes *in addition* to any struggles we have in our interactions with the health care system on account of sexism, racism, class, age or disability. It is not surprising that so many of us feel unable to be open about our sexuality when seeking health care. In one large British survey almost 68 per cent of lesbians were not out even to their GP, while the Michigan Lesbian Health Survey reported that 61 per cent of lesbians felt unable to come out to any health care provider.[15] Indeed, a substantial minority of lesbians, when questioned about their experiences of health care, describe health care situations as dangerous: they feared they might be harmed in health care interactions if they became known as lesbians; some felt safe only when accompanied by a partner or friend who could act as a witness or advocate.[16]
>
> Worryingly, it seems that many of us will go to great lengths to avoid interactions with the health care system. This has obvious consequences for our health. Lesbians are less likely to seek regular routine care (such as cervical smear testing or breast examination) which might pick up potential problems at an early stage, are more likely to put up with worrying symptoms until they become unmanageable and are more likely to regard the formal health care system as a last resort.[17] There are some benefits of our tendency to stay away from doctors at all costs – for example we are probably less likely to be given unnecessary treatment – but these are far outweighed by the risks to our health which come when we delay seeking help for possibly serious conditions which medical science may be able to deal with.

Defiance in the face of doctors:
being a successful patient

An added factor which makes going to the doctor more difficult for many lesbians than for non-lesbian women is simply that we are less accustomed to doctors. Most lesbians have fewer reasons to seek health care on a routine basis, simply because we do not have sex with men. Having sex with men means two things – contraception and pregnancy – which require women to get involved with health care services on a very intimate level. From adolescence, most heterosexually active women have to get used to doctors, nurses and clinic staff asking intimate questions about their sexual behaviour, peering into their vaginas, taking blood samples, monitoring blood pressure, feeling their breasts and taking cervical smears or vaginal swabs. The successful management of reproductive heterosexuality requires a woman to submit herself to a range of medical interventions in a way which is just not necessary for women who don't have sex with men. Heterosexual women don't *like* all this business – in fact they complain about it all the time, but after a while you just have to get used to it.

❝ *I was heterosexual for years, and I've been married. During this time I got used to regular gynaecological examinations for contraception, recurrent cystitis, pre-natal care and a variety of infections. When I became a lesbian, all this attention stopped overnight. I now hardly ever see a doctor. I had to have an internal examination recently, and I must admit it really did feel strange to have my doctor put her fingers inside my vagina. After all, that's a big part of my sex life now!* ❞

'Lesley'

There are suggestions on how you can make the experience of an internal examination less unpleasant later in this chapter (pp. 206–8), but how can lesbians ensure that *all* our interactions with health care services are positive ones?

Dealing with doctors: whose health are we talking about here?

In the industrialized West, women are brought up to be polite and considerate and not to make a fuss. When you are dealing with experts, whether they are brain surgeons or garage mechanics, this is not a helpful approach. One of the early insights of feminism was that assertiveness, rather than ladylike politeness, was essential to women's survival in a male-dominated world. Feminist research has shown that it is very hard for women to get their health care needs taken seriously, and that being polite and well-behaved can put women at a real disadvantage in our interactions with the health care system.[18] For lesbians, this problem may be even more acute, since during any health care consultation we may be putting effort either into concealing our sexuality or into monitoring the consequences of disclosing it. If it does not feel safe or appropriate to be out during a consultation, we may be unwilling to make a fuss or to be stubborn, in order to get out of an unsafe situation as quickly as possible. If we have come out, we may feel grateful that the other person accepts this information or we may feel angry and upset if they respond inappropriately. In either case, being a troublesome patient/client is not going to feel like a good strategy!

It is hard enough to argue with a plumber or a car mechanic if you suspect you are receiving poor service from them. But doctors have, as a profession, managed to get themselves into a position of high social status and very real power, and it can be a struggle not to be intimidated by them. In addition, you are likely to be feeling concerned and vulnerable (or you wouldn't be seeing the doctor in the first place) and they do have certain powers which have direct consequences for your health. They may refuse to treat you, may blind you with medical jargon, or may label you 'difficult', 'neurotic' or even 'mentally unstable'. When these labels are applied by medical professionals, they have real sticking power, and may have an effect on the kind of health care we receive in consequence. But the power is not all with doctors. They may be in a powerful position, but they also have clearly defined responsibilities, and you have rights.

The first step to getting good health care is to be absolutely clear about what you are doing in seeking professional help. When you visit a doctor – whether they are paid by the state or work privately – their salary in the long run comes out of your pocket. They have chosen to do the job they are doing because it meets their idea of what a good job is, and they have undertaken to provide the best service possible to everyone who seeks their professional advice. *It is their job to provide you with effective and impartial professional services.* If they haven't taken the trouble to educate themselves about lesbian health issues, or if they are rude or offensive to their lesbian clients, they are not doing their job well. There are a few steps you can take to make sure that you get the best service possible from your doctor.

- If possible, seek out health care from practitioners who are firmly located in the lesbian community or who are known to be lesbian-friendly. Go to a lesbian clinic, ask your lesbian friends for a recommendation, or ring your local lesbian and gay switchboard or help-line and ask if they can recommend anyone.

- Very few doctors are well informed about lesbians or about our health needs. The better informed you are, the more information you can bring to the consultation.

- Most professionals find it difficult to admit that there are major gaps in their knowledge, or that their professional practice is not up to scratch. Be prepared to share *your* knowledge in a gentle and non-aggressive manner (even if you feel like screaming).

- Educate yourself about how your local health care system works, and especially what support you can expect if things go wrong. In Britain, check out your local Community Health Council (some have more teeth than others) or Citizens' Advice Bureau; in the USA or Canada find out about local advocacy groups or lesbian/gay health organizations (see Further Reading section). Support may be forthcoming from your trade union or other professional body.

- Find out about alternative or complementary practitioners who offer services in your area. These may be more expensive than mainstream services, and of course many are just as ignorant about lesbians. But many such practitioners are informed of issues around sexuality, and many may themselves be lesbian, gay or feminist.

- Don't assume that a mainstream doctor is going to be a raving homophobe until s/he gives you reason to think this. There are as many lesbians in medicine, nursing and the professions allied to medicine as there are in any other part of the workforce, and many non-lesbian health care workers are genuinely concerned to provide good services to their lesbian clients.

I am not suggesting that you approach every consultation with a briefcase full of medical ethics textbooks in your hand and a solicitor peeping over your shoulder to record evidence of malpractice. But if you know as much as you can about your rights, the support services available to you and alternative forms of care, you will feel much stronger when dealing with doctors and will be much less daunted in your consultations with them.

To be out to your doctor or not: that is the question

Only you can decide whether or not to come out to the health care professionals you deal with. We all know that the experience of coming out is not something which you do once in your life and never have to do again. Lesbians have to make decisions about coming out on a daily basis, and it never ends. You may come out for very different reasons to different people – there may be absolutely nothing to be gained by telling the postman, the plumber or the baker but every reason to tell your boss, your parents or the solicitor handling your child custody case. There are certainly very good reasons why it might be particularly important for your doctor to have accurate information about your sexuality. If both of you mean completely different things when you use the word 'sex', or if your insomnia or high blood pressure is due to you being harassed at work, then the fact that you are a lesbian has a bearing on the kind of care your doctor should be providing. If you are one of a couple receiving care from a midwife during pregnancy and birth, then you will probably want to ensure that the non-biological co-mother is recognized and treated as such, and not just as a special friend.

You may also need to ensure that your partner is recognized as your next of kin if you are hospitalized, and this requires that you make the nature of your relationship explicit.

The same may or may not be true of any other health care staff you come into contact with: nurses, physiotherapists, health visitors, etc. It is important to keep in control of the extent to which your sexual identity is known in a health care situation, and you can best do this by making it clear to each person you choose to tell that the information is confidential and you do not want it to be passed on. If you do not want your sexuality to be on your medical records, you should make this quite clear at every stage.

> 66 *I told them I was a lesbian and once, when I was waiting in Outpatients, I had a look at my record. And there it was, written on my record, 'lesbian'. I was really angry, there was no way I wanted everyone I came into contact with to have that information about me. But I was too scared to ask them to take it off.* 99

'Janet'

It is not only medical professionals who may have very negative or hostile attitudes to lesbians. Many of us use the services of complementary or alternative practitioners – homoeopaths, acupuncturists, reflexologists, herbalists, etc. – and, although we may expect that people working in these traditions are more open minded and informed, this is not necessarily the case.

> 66 *I had found therapeutic massage very helpful, and wanted to treat my then partner to a session. The masseuse assured me that 'I can see* him *on any weekday'. I gently corrected her, telling her my partner was a woman. She apologised profusely, saying that she should not have made assumptions, but she was completely different with me from that moment. She was clearly uncomfortable with massaging me, and it got so tense that I had to give up going to her. That was dreadful, she was one of the best masseuses I have been to.* 99

'Max'

So being open about your sexuality may lead to difficulties, but it is almost certainly better than remaining in the closet. Not only is it difficult to ensure that you get appropriate care if you pass as heterosexual, but it also takes a lot of energy which you could otherwise be using to deal effectively with your health problem and is in itself stressful. It is also important to remember that the more lesbians come out to health care professionals, the less able those professionals are to convince themselves they have never met a lesbian, and the more likely it is that lesbian health care needs will be taken seriously. I am not asking you to be a martyr for the cause of lesbian sisterhood, but if you do decide to be out in your dealings with the health care system, you can congratulate yourself that you are making life easier for lesbians coming after you.

What services do lesbians need?

Lesbians need exactly the same from health care providers as anyone else does. We need full and easy access to *primary care*, the regular health checks and tests that enable us to spot potentially serious problems soon enough to have them treated effectively. We need full and easy access to emergency treatment when we are injured or acutely ill (sometimes called *secondary care*). We need good-quality and effective ante-natal and midwifery care if and when we choose to have children. We need good-quality and effective social care in emergencies: for example, homelessness, rape, bereavement, domestic violence or recovery from substance addiction. We need good and effective services to support us in maintaining full emotional and mental health and in recovering our emotional and mental wellbeing at times of crisis. All these services need to be developed in full recognition of the specific needs which we may have because we are lesbians, and should be provided to us with respect and sensitivity. When seeking help from the health and social care professions, every lesbian should expect to be treated with awareness and respect by people who have a good level of knowledge about the issues which she is dealing with *as a lesbian*. If this does not happen, it is a failure on the part of the professional, *not* the responsibility of the lesbian concerned!

Sailing through internal examinations

This section aims to demystify some of the health care procedures which should be routinely available to all of us. For a lesbian, especially if she has never had penetrative sex with a man, the internal examination which is such a routine part of gynaecological health care can be very distressing. Yet such examinations are a useful and important part of lesbian health care. We are *not* immune to cancers of the cervix, vagina, uterus or ovaries, and an internal examination with cervical smear (called 'pap smear' in the USA) should be a routine way of looking after ourselves. So what can you do to make it less of an ordeal?

The first thing is to know what will happen. Many health problems that affect the ovaries, uterus, vagina, bladder or cervix don't cause any noticeable problems in the early stages, or may cause symptoms which are easily dismissed as wind or other trivial causes. So a full internal examination will check all these organs. The person who examines you will wear sterile latex gloves, which will not have been used on anyone else and which will be thrown away after they have been used on you. These gloves are very thin and sensitive, and should not cause you any discomfort.[19] By inserting two fingers of one hand into your vagina, and by gentle pressure on your abdomen and pelvic region with the other hand, the person examining you will be able to feel the size, shape and position of your uterus and ovaries. This will feel strange – it is an odd sensation having someone you hardly know rummage around inside you – but should not be painful. If you remind yourself that valuable information about your health is being obtained by this relatively easy process, it becomes easier to relax. It is helpful if you breathe slowly and deeply and concentrate on relaxing the muscles of your stomach, rather than tensing up.

At some point a *speculum* will be used, in order to make a visual inspection of your vagina and cervix and to take a cervical smear and any swabs that are needed. This is the bit which many women dislike most, but it doesn't have to be unpleasant. When closed, a speculum is designed to slide easily into your vagina. Once inside, it can be opened using a screw mechanism, in order to part the

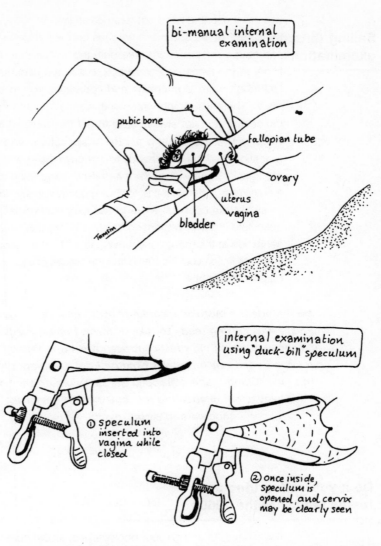

bi-manual internal examination

pubic bone

fallopian tube

ovary

uterus

vagina

bladder

Tamsin

internal examination using "duck-bill" speculum

① speculum inserted into vagina while closed

② once inside, speculum is opened, and cervix may be clearly seen

walls of the vagina and bring your cervix into view, so that a smear may be taken. The smear itself is taken by gently passing a specially designed wooden spatula across the neck of the womb. You will feel pressure, since the whole object of the exercise is to remove a few cells from the cervix for examination, but it should not hurt. If you feel pain when the speculum is opened, this may be for one of two reasons; either the speculum is being opened too fast when you are tense and have not been given time to relax, or sometimes the 'beak' of the speculum catches on the cervix as it opens. This can cause quite a sharp little pain (no worse than catching your finger in the hinge of a small box, but in the circumstances it can feel much more frightening), and can cause you to clench up and resist. There is nothing wrong with saying 'Ouch! I think you've hit my cervix!' It is not always easy to get the cervix in the right place when you are operating a vaginal speculum, and a competent practitioner will be quite happy to withdraw the speculum gently and start again. *It really should not hurt if it is being done correctly: if you feel pain it is a sign that it is not being done properly*. Once the smear or swab has been taken, and the examination is complete, the speculum is gently withdrawn, still open. This can cause a stretching sensation at the mouth of your vagina, but if the speculum is closed while still inside you, it could pinch the tissues of your vagina, possibly causing bruising.

> 66 *I made the mistake of coming out to the practice nurse when she was getting ready to take a smear. I had my legs open, and she was asking me what contraceptives I use. When I told her I don't need contraceptives because I am a lesbian, I heard this loud 'Clang!'. She'd dropped the speculum on the floor. She was not offensive to me, but she was obviously shocked and embarrassed.* 99
>
> 'Elizabeth'

Do it yourself: a tried and tested legacy of the 1960s

If you have, lurking on your bookshelves, an old copy of the feminist bestseller *Our Bodies Ourselves*, you will recall that the authors suggest purchasing your own speculum and getting used to examining your own cervix. This is not for everyone, but it is not difficult, and it can make going for routine smear tests a much less fraught experience. You can buy a cheap plastic speculum from most medical suppliers, or you may be able to get one from your local women's clinic or well woman centre. You may want to splash out on a steel one; these are identical to the ones which health professionals will be using when they examine you, and will last you a lifetime. Mine has been in regular use since 1980 and is still gleaming like new.

Once you have purchased your speculum, make some private time to get used to using it. Warm it up with warm water (*don't* make it too hot!) and use plenty of KY jelly around the entrance to your vagina and smeared on the beak of the speculum to ease insertion. I find it easiest to use a speculum sitting up on a bed with my back supported, but you may find it easier lying on your back, or even standing up. Remember those little diagrams in the tampon boxes, which caused such anxiety when you were first practising? It's a bit like that all over again. Practise opening and locking the speculum *before* inserting it for the first time. Once it is in place, gently start turning the screw mechanism until is is as wide open as is comfortable. You may find that you have caught your cervix in the wrong place, which will cause a minor, but sharp, pain. If this happens, gently withdraw the speculum *still in the open position*, close it and start again. It takes a bit of practice to get it right, but once you have speculum, torch and mirror in the right place, you will see your cervix. It is exciting to be looking at this significant part of your body, which is normally visible only to medical professionals. Once you are able to use a speculum with confidence, there is nothing to prevent you taking charge during gynaecological examinations – try taking your own speculum along and asking if you can insert it yourself. Keep it clean between examinations using hot soapy water. As you become familiar with how your cervix looks and the changes that take place at various points in your menstrual cycle or over a lifetime, you may be alerted to changes which are abnormal for you. For more information about what to look at when doing self-examination, contact your local women's health group or consult *Our Bodies Ourselves*.

When someone else's hand is on the speculum

It helps to know that speculums come in many sizes, as indeed do vaginas. Many doctors and nurses assume that adult women regularly experience vaginal penetration by a penis and that they can accommodate a large speculum. For many lesbians, who may not include penetration in their sexual practices or who may never have been penetrated by anything larger than a finger, this may be inappropriate.

> 66 *Eventually I gave in and had a smear test, but it was awful, really painful. Once was enough, I'm never going to have one again.* 99

'Dale'

There is absolutely no reason why you shouldn't say to the person examining you 'Please use a small speculum.' You should also ask that they warm it first (the feeling of cold chrome would be enough to make Mae West a little tense!), and that plenty of lubricant is used. A competent doctor or nurse will do all these things as a matter of course (and courtesy), but it is in your interests to make sure they do. After all, it's your vagina!

You should make sure that you get a regular cervical smear test, although there is little agreement among doctors about just how often smears should be done. Averaging out many conflicting recommendations it seems likely that getting a smear every two or three years is probably the best course to take, unless your doctor or health care worker advises you differently. But please remember that many health care professionals still believe that lesbians are not at risk from cervical cancer and that we do not need regular smears. *This is not the case*, and you should not allow a doctor to persuade you that you do not need smears.

Other regular tests and check-ups

As well as regular smears, there are other tests which should be done regularly. You may want to examine your own breasts regularly (although there is some disagreement about the usefulness of regular self-examination) and to keep an eye on your blood pressure. Heterosexually active women have their blood pressure checked as part of regular care if they are taking the contraceptive pill, and lesbians are less likely to have hypertension picked up in this routine way. It is a good idea to have your blood pressure tested once a year, and for your doctor to get an idea of what is a normal range for you. People's blood pressure does vary, and a high reading does not necessarily mean you need treatment. Some minority ethnic groups are at particular risk of hypertension – it is a silent killer of many African-American women for example – and since it is associated with stress, there are reasons to suspect that it might be a particular issue for lesbians (although I am aware of no research which has been done in this area).

You may wish to consider a mammogram – a breast X-ray – as a way of detecting breast cancer at an early stage. In Britain, women are invited for a regular mammogram once they reach the age of fifty, and cancer specialists sometimes recommend that women with a history of breast cancer in the family should receive mammograms before this age. However, dosing the healthy breast with radiation is *not* a good idea, since any dose of radiation carries a health risk. You may wish to put your faith in self-examination, and leave more technological investigations to be called upon if you find any suspicious changes. Many centres now use ultrasound, which carries no known risks. If you are worried about the effects of radiation on your body, you could try asking if ultrasound is available in your area.

To examine your breasts, choose the same time each month (even if you have stopped menstruating). The breast is not just a lump of flesh, it is a complex and dynamic organ which changes constantly, and your breasts are less full and easier to examine just after your period has stopped. First, have a good look at your breasts while you are standing in front of a mirror. Check for any *change* in outline, in skin texture (especially puckering or dimpling of the skin), in the position of your nipples or in the nipples themselves. Gently squeeze your nipples and check for any unusual discharge (some women have a light discharge at certain times of their cycle, and you will know if this is usual for you). Then lie down on a flat surface and examine each breast in turn with the opposite hand, putting the other arm behind your head. Don't poke at your breast or knead it with the tips of your fingers, but make smooth circular movements outwards from the nipple, using the *flat* of your fingers and gentle pressure. Extend this right up into the armpit. You will feel all kinds of bumps and gristly tissue at first, and this may be alarming if you are not used to the feel of your breasts. The key here is symmetry. Something which you can feel in the same place in both breasts is normal for you.

If you do find something which you think is suspicious, you will almost cetainly feel scared and panicky. This is only to be expected: after all, there has been a great deal of publicity about breast cancer in the lesbian community recently. But remember, the vast majority of lumps turn out to be completely harmless. You will not be putting yourself at risk if you wait for four or five weeks before seeing a doctor. If the lump shrinks, vanishes or moves to a different location during this time, it is not cancer and you may decide that no further examination is necessary. However, if you are extremely anxious or scared, and you feel unable to wait for a few weeks, do consult your doctor and ask them to do a full breast examination. Many doctors nowadays will refer a woman with a breast lump for a second opinion. *This does not mean that your doctor thinks you have cancer*, it is simply a responsible way of ensuring that there is no possible room for misdiagnosis.

Further tests, including ultrasound, needle aspiration, manual examination or biopsy, may be used to confirm a diagnosis. If you have reason to be concerned about the possibility of contracting breast cancer, or if you have been told that you have the disease, it is useful to find out as much as you can from as many sources as you can so that you can be actively involved in any steps taken to safeguard your health. *The New Our Bodies Ourselves* (see Further Reading) has an extensive section on breast disease.

Getting the best out of complementary healing traditions

A few decades ago, few people questioned medical wisdom. Doctors, it was generally believed, know what is good for you. In Britain, where the first national health service was set up, this feeling was mixed with pride and gratitude as ordinary people took advantage of services which were available to them for the first time ever. Nowadays this euphoria about scientific medicine has faded. As it becomes clear that there are limits to modern medicine – that it cannot yet cure the common cold, that it is unable to contain the

HIV pandemic, that doctors are as fallible and corrupt as anyone else – more and more people are beginning to question their dependence on doctors. What is more, medical 'advances' have led to a whole new set of problems. The indiscriminate use of antibiotics has resulted in new strains of bacteria developing resistance. New infections are appearing in hospitals, proving extremely difficult to eradicate and making some patients more gravely ill than they were when they were admitted. Most treatments, especially those involving drugs or irradiation, have side effects which can be more damaging than the initial problem, and for some terminal conditions the drive to prolong life at any cost can mean that the last few weeks of a person's life are spent undergoing unpleasant and miserable 'treatments' rather than preparing for the end of life. Increasingly, doubts are being voiced about whether scientific medical treatment should be unthinkingly trusted with our wellbeing. More and more people are turning to other healing traditions, some of them – such as acupuncture – much older than modern medicine, others – like homoeopathy – of more recent origin.

For lesbians, using alternative or complementary practitioners may be especially appealing. Such practitioners are, like lesbians, somewhat outside the mainstream of society. They have, by definition, questioned the values of that mainstream, and might therefore be expected to have a more open and accepting approach to sexuality. In addition, women tend to be better represented among the ranks of complementary practitioners, and there is not the same hierarchical structure that dogs the medical profession. Many lesbian feminists may perceive women acupuncturists, herbalists, homoeopaths and other practitioners as continuing an unbroken tradition of women healers which the full might of patriarchal power (in the form of the Catholic Inquisition and later the male-dominated medical establishment) has been unable to stamp out.

It is difficult to generalize about lesbians as a group, since we are all many things as well as being lesbians. There are undoubtedly large numbers of lesbians whose treatment of choice is, and will remain, scientific medicine. However, research does seem to indicate that lesbians are more inclined to question the practices of modern medicine, and that we are more likely to want to use alternative healing traditions:

Being unsatisfied with the current Western medical approaches of medication and surgery [lesbians] sought alternative health practices that are less invasive and more in tune with the human body and nature.[20]

Dissatisfaction with Western medicine is one thing, finding an alternative that works for you is another. After all, there are hundreds of different treatments on offer, from those which have been proved over thousands of years to hare-brained schemes dreamed up by optimistic and charismatic individuals with a tenuous hold on reality or ethics. How do you tell the difference?

It is important to know the limitations of the different traditions on offer, and to recognize when the resources of medical science can be usefully integrated with more beneficial healing methods. For example, one thing which Western medicine is pretty good at (at least in theory) is diagnosis. If, for example, you have a tumour in your bowel, it may be identified faster with up-to-date imaging techniques than by the painstaking questioning of an alternative practitioner. However, this assumes that your doctor recognizes the symptoms you present him or her with and takes you and the symptoms seriously, and that you have access to diagnostic equipment and the people with the knowledge to operate it. In theory, all this should be available to you within a state-funded national health care system. If you don't have state-funded health care and you lack private insurance or your insurance doesn't cover the tests you need, then you may simply not have access to the diagnostic strengths of modern medicine anyway. If you do, then you may decide to make use of them and then, armed with your diagnosis, decide what combination of various healing options to make use of. Not easy to do at the best of times, and very difficult when you are stressed out and not thinking very clearly because you are ill or worried.

It is probably a good idea to find out about what is available in your area *before* you need it. Ask friends and colleagues about their experiences with various alternative health care traditions and keep a note of the name and address of any practitioner who comes highly recommended. Make sure you know who is and who is not lesbian-aware and lesbian-friendly. By all means support practitioners who are themselves lesbian, but be aware of possible problems. I once found myself in a very tricky situation involving a somewhat

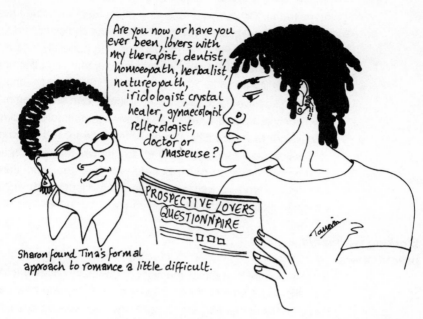

Sharon found Tina's formal
approach to romance a little difficult.

unprofessional lesbian homoeopath and a recent ex-lover. It ended
with me convinced that a lover is just a lover, but a good homoeopath
should be for life. Boundaries need to be carefully maintained in
small lesbian communities, and this can complicate matters for the
clients of lesbian practitioners.

Another source of information about complementary healing
traditions is books. Your local community bookshop is probably
bursting at the seams with guides to complementary medicine. It is
well worth investing in a good general guide which will give you some
idea of how homoeopathy works, how to check out the credentials
of your local herbalist, etc. Some such guides are listed in the Further
Reading section, but there are far too many to list here and new
ones are published every year. It is also a good idea, if you are
interested in trying out a particular treatment, to find out how
practitioners are trained, what qualifications they need and how their
conduct is governed. If you write off to a central regulating body,
such as the Society of Homoeopaths or the Shiatsu Society or (for
more general inquiries) the Council for Complementary and Alternative
Medicine (in Britain), you will be able to get lists of registered

practitioners, and information about the kinds of treatment you are interested in. Or visit your local complementary or natural healing clinic. These are mushrooming in major towns and cities throughout Europe, Australasia and North America, and generally hold stocks of informative leaflets about the various treatments on offer, or even a reference library.

Once you have decided to try a particular form of treatment, and have chosen a practitioner, make an arrangement for a preliminary discussion. Most practitioners do not charge for this. During this discussion, you should be able to assess whether this particular treatment is likely to be of benefit, whether the practitioner is comfortable working with lesbian clients, and (at the simplest level) whether you like and feel that you can trust her or him.

Working with male practitioners

If it is important to you that you work only with a woman practitioner, you should be able to track one down, although you may have to range a little further afield to do so. Many men working in alternative health care are wonderful – I had regular Shiatsu sessions with a male practitioner for years, and he was respectful, committed and delightful – but some seem to think that working as a healer is enough on its own to make the fact that they are men irrelevant. They can get quite cross if women still treat them as if they were 'ordinary' men. But of course there *are* alternative practitioners who oppress or abuse women clients, and being a nice, gentle bearded man in a hand-knitted jumper is not enough to reverse centuries of patriarchal oppression or to reassure a woman who has suffered rape or abuse. Any man who thinks it is should not, perhaps, be the first-choice health care practitioner for lesbians.

Paying for alternative health care

It is possible that the state or your health insurance will pay for alternative treatment. Certainly some fundholding general practices in Britain are happy to pay for their patients to receive acupuncture, homoeopathy, therapeutic massage or some other forms of treatment. Not only do some doctors recognize the benefits of such treatments, but also they are likely to be cheaper than drugs or in-patient care. However, it is more likely that you will *not* be able to get your treatment of choice paid for. It may be worth setting aside a small savings fund to enable you to pay for private complementary treatment if and when you need to. A small sum paid each week into a savings account is a realistic option for many lesbians (though not those struggling to survive on most state benefits). Or you could sign up for a short-term insurance policy which will pay out a lump sum if you become sick, and use those funds to pay for any alternative treatments you may need.

Longer-term issues:
getting good treatment in hospitals

It is one thing being assertive enough to demand and get good-quality services from your doctor or alternative health care provider. It is very different getting good care during a hospital stay. For a start, if you are ill enough to require hospital treatment, you are likely to be vulnerable and concerned. So, indeed, are those close to you, your family, partner or friends. Then there is the nature of hospital care, which tends to be fragmented and stressful. Surprising numbers of people are responsible for your wellbeing while you are in hospital, from dieticians, cooks, laundry workers, radiographers, surgeons and cleaners to nurses, physiotherapists, pathologists, social workers and porters. Most of them you will not even meet. Those most directly involved in your care will be your medical team and the nursing staff. Nurses in particular have the power to make your stay comfortable and relaxed or utterly miserable. Unfortunately, survey after survey reveals high levels of homophobia among nurses, linked in particular to strong religious beliefs.[21] Nurses have been disrespectful to lesbian patients, their lesbian friends or their partners, and have in some cases failed to provide an adequate standard of care.[22]

Nursing has historically tended to be a conservative occupation, although more recent developments towards professionalizing nursing have resulted in some very real changes. Some nursing bodies, for example the Royal College of Nursing (RCN) in England, promote very radical policies aimed at ensuring that the best possible nursing care is available to lesbians and gay men. In March 1994 the RCN issued a formal statement, *The Nursing Care of Lesbians and Gay Men*, in which it described a general failure of the profession to meet the needs of this client group, and set out a strategy to remedy this. The opening paragraphs set the tone:

The Royal College of Nursing recognizes through work undertaken by its members that discrimination and prejudice towards lesbian and gay patients exists in nursing.

This statement outlines the RCN's commitment to developing and promoting good nursing practice for this group of clients and to the support and assistance of any nurses who experience difficulties in developing their practice in this area.

It is very important for nurses to have the formal support of the RCN in this way, and it is useful for lesbians who are going into hospital to know that the RCN recognizes the nursing needs of lesbians, and that there is a professional expectation that nurses will treat lesbian clients properly. Where such support is absent from professional bodies, the job of individual practitioners is much more difficult, and the position of lesbian patients or clients is less powerful.

Whether you, as a lesbian about to enter hospital, are able to ensure that you receive a high standard of nursing care should not depend solely on the policies of nursing bodies. There are some steps you can take to make life easier for yourself. If you have a partner you will want her to have all the rights which heterosexual partners receive as a matter of course. These include visiting rights, which may be particularly important if you are going to spend time in intensive care; the right to obtain accurate information about your health and your progress over the telephone or in person; the right to be present during intimate examinations if you so desire; and the right to be consulted over your treatment if you become too ill to make decisions on your own behalf. Since lesbian partnerships are not automatically recognized by the law in many countries, it may be worth your while getting legal advice so that you can enshrine your and your partner's wishes in a legal contract. Depending on the country you live in, and on the circumstances, you may wish to make a living will, or to give your lover power of attorney (in Canada, Medical Power of Attorney), or simply to name her formally as your next of kin. None of these is foolproof, any may be contested by your blood relatives, but they do have some status in the eyes of hospital staff. You should be able to get advice on finding a lesbian-friendly solicitor (some of whom give their services free in community law centres) from your local lesbian and gay switchboard, helpline or community group. Another useful avenue can be AIDS voluntary groups, since they have plenty of experience in dealing with same-sex relationships in the context of serious illness and hospitalization. They may also have their own legal team or friendly volunteer legal expert who may be able to give you some basic advice free over the telephone.

All this talk about legal contracts and homophobic nurses can make it seem as if staying in hospital will be a battle from start to finish. This is not necessarily the case. There are instances of lesbians being poorly treated by nursing staff, but nurses are an extremely overworked group of people, and for most people (not just lesbians) the fantasy of the cool hand on the fevered brow vanishes when confronted with the realities of hospital life. Nurses are rushed off their feet, shift changes mean that you will see a stream of new faces, and it is all too easy to interpret the brusqueness of a tired or distracted nurse as a sign that she hates lesbians when in fact the causes are much simpler! The majority of lesbians have no worse a time in hospital than anyone else. If you go in already defensive and hostile, expecting trouble and prepared to fight for your rights, you may not be the easiest person in the world to nurse. If you are friendly and open, and behave as though you expect people to be friendly and open with you, you will soon spot whether you have been unlucky enough to get landed with a genuinely homophobic nurse. If that happens, keep notes for a day or two about any incidents which seem to you to be evidence of discriminatory treatment, and get your visitors to keep their own notes. Then ask to speak to the nurse in charge of your ward, and discuss the issue quietly with them.

Apart from possible troubles with homophobic staff, the key to surviving a hospital stay is to prepare as well as possible. If you are going in for an operation under general anaesthetic, be aware that it can take your body weeks to fully excrete the anaesthetic drugs, and that during that time you may feel depressed, fatigued or just vaguely unwell. For a couple of days after an operation, especially if it is a lengthy one, you will feel sore, bruised and not up to entertaining huge numbers of visitors. Take a survival pack into hospital with you to make your body feel loved and cared for – your favourite treats in the form of chocolate, fruit, fruit juices or other small goodies, an indulgent bath oil or hand-made soap, enough clean pyjamas so that you don't have to put up with the same ones for too long, your favourite massage oil or body rub, and comfortable slippers. You may feel less like reading than you imagine, so now is *not* the time to get stuck into that learned book of feminist theory which has been gathering dust on your shelves for years. Take a new novel by a favourite writer and some favourite tapes for your personal stereo. You may find sleeping difficult (especially since you may be woken up very early in the morning), so you may wish to take ear plugs and an eye mask for daytime naps. Consult your complementary practitioner about the treatment you will be receiving, and see if there is anything which will help your recovery. Homoeopathic doses of arnica montana, for example, can dramatically reduce bruising and pain from an operation and can help general recovery. Above all, make sure that you are able to relax and not worry about the responsibilities you have left behind you. If your child(ren), pets, pot plants and garden are being well looked after, now is the time to take a break from feeling responsible for them.

What about the children?

If you are going to have to spend time in hospital, your child(ren) will quite naturally be anxious. But this need not be traumatic for them. Make sure they know who will be taking care of them, when they can come and visit you, and what to expect when they do. If possible, take them to visit the hospital before you are admitted, so that the building is not completely unfamiliar and they have time to get used to the noise, the size, the lights and the smell. It's not a bad idea for you to get used to these things too! If you can afford it, buy a small toy or book to take in with you, so that when they come to visit, you can give them something to focus their attention on other than how poorly you seem. Make sure that your medical team and nursing staff know that your child(ren) will be coming in. Explain to your child(ren) what is going to happen to you in terms that they can understand, and try to prepare them for the fact that you may be sleepy, or may be speaking very quietly or slowly, and that this is nothing to worry about. Make sure that whoever brings them to visit you at hospital is able to comfort them if they become worried or upset, and arrange with hospital staff if you want your child(ren) to have unrestricted contact with you by telephone. If you are prepared to be woken at four in the morning to talk to an upset child who needs to be reassured that you are OK, then make that clear to whoever is caring for the child(ren) and to the hospital staff.

As a lesbian mother, you will be familiar with the feeling that your mothering is constantly under scrutiny, and that you have to be a supermum in order to deflect homophobic criticism. Having your kids visit you in hospital may spark off those feelings. Just remember that *all* kids seem out of place in an adult ward, and that the staff have much better things to do than concern themselves with any imagined inadequacies in your mothering!

The limits to health care

It is important to understand that regular health checks and the best health care in the world do not make anyone healthy. Such checks give us potentially valuable information about our health but that is *all* that they do, whilst medical treatment can help us recover from illness, but it cannot necessarily prevent illness or make us positively healthy. Some women, for example, believe that, until the treatment for breast cancer is greatly improved, they would rather not have mammograms, since the benefits of an early diagnosis of breast cancer are unclear. Others would rather know as soon as possible, so that they may direct their energies to fighting the disease.

How to be a lesbian health activist

The causes of ill health are complex, but we can be sure that *all* causes of ill health, from accidents to disease, are more likely to affect people who are socially disadvantaged. Of course it is useful for individual lesbians to be able to demand appropriate health care services as and when needed, and to have the information necessary to make positive choices to safeguard health and wellbeing. But it is becoming increasingly clear that health is more closely associated with *social* factors than with anything else.[23] This means that anyone who is interested in improving the health of themselves and other lesbians needs to become a health activist.

If you want to become a lesbian health activist, you may want get together with other lesbians. This will ensure that you get support, and will also prevent you reinventing the wheel (since activity may already be going on in the area you are interested in) so check out lesbian groups in your area. The Lesbian Avengers, ACTUP and other organizations may have local groups working on lesbian health (the London chapter of the Lesbian Avengers recently produced a leaflet for lesbians on breast cancer, for example), and local feminist health groups may be interested in pursuing lesbian issues.[24] If you are concerned about a single issue – HIV/AIDS or breast cancer for example – get in touch with organizations which campaign around that issue and see if they have a lesbian section or if they would like you to start one. An alternative approach is to get involved in the wider community and put lesbian health on the agenda there. In England and Wales, get yourself elected on to the local Community Health Council or the user's group of your GP practice (if there isn't one, suggest starting one). In the USA or Canada, join a local community health group or citizens' advocacy group and lobby for lesbian health issues in that forum. When issues such as lesbian adoption or partnership rights come into the public eye, as they do from time to time, write to your MP, Senator or Euro MP expressing your views on the matter and asking for their support in any forthcoming legislation. Write to local and national newspapers – why should the bigots be the only ones whose voices get heard?

If you are yourself a health care professional, or if you are involved in the education and training of health care professionals, there will be many steps you can take, both large and small, to ensure that lesbian health gets taken seriously. There are also steps you can take to ensure that lesbian clients get a better service. Even something as simple as bringing your old copies of *Diva*, *Curve* or other community publications in to add to the pile of reading material in clinic waiting rooms will send a powerful signal to lesbian clients that someone, somewhere, recognizes that they exist. No clinic, hospital, surgery or practice anywhere should be without a poster on its public noticeboard listing the local numbers of lesbian and gay helplines and social groups. If it gets torn down, put a fresh one up. If someone complains, welcome the opportunity for a little consciousness-raising.

Improving lesbian health, and getting good health care services for all lesbians, is a massive task. It requires some pretty major shifts in social attitudes, and it requires the medical and health care professions to recognize an area where their practice to date has been unprofessional and to do something about that. But there is ample evidence that these shifts are starting to happen, and every positive action, whether it be a big one like successfully lobbying to defeat discriminatory legislation or a small one like anonymously sticking lesbian helpline numbers on the backs of doors in women's toilets, helps to speed the progress of change.

Further reading

There is not much available from a specifically lesbian perspective, but all these books contain useful material.

Regan McClure and Anne Vespry (eds), *Lesbian Health Guide* (Toronto: Queer Press, 1994). Has a good section on getting the best possible care, although much of it is specific to Canada.

Boston Women's Health Book Collective (eds), *The New Our Bodies Ourselves* (Harmondsworth: Penguin, 1989). The best source of comprehensive advice and information about health care services.

Peggy Foster, *Women and the Health Care Industry: An Unhealthy Relationship?* (Milton Keynes: Open University Press, 1995). A useful feminist critique of the health care system, but has nothing about lesbians and is untrustworthy in the area of HIV/AIDS.

Carolyn Faulder, *Whose Body Is It? The Troubling Issue of Informed Consent* (London: Virago, 1985). A feminist discussion of this basic doctor/patient issue.

Susan Curtis and Romy Fraser, *Natural Healing for Women: Caring for Yourself with Herbs, Homoeopathy and Essential Oils* (London: Pandora, 1995). A useful self-help guide.

Rina Nissim, *Natural Healing in Gynaecology: A Manual for Women* (London: Pandora, 1996). A useful self-help guide.

Anne Woodham, *HEA Guide to Complementary Medicine and Therapies* (London: Health Education Authority, 1994). A clear introductory guide to the complicated world of alternative health care.

Notes

Notes to Introduction

1. From Miriam Stoppard's book *Being a Well Woman: How to Achieve and Maintain Personal Fitness, Health and Happiness* (New York: Holt, Rinehart and Winston, 1982), p. 403.
2. Stoppard not only fails to recognize the existence of lesbians, but she refuses to address any woman who isn't white. Suggesting that black women 'blanch' (i.e., whiten) their skin is grotesque and racist.
3. Stoppard (note 1), pp. 86–7

Notes to Chapter 1

1. This is not as odd as it sounds. Medical science has been hard at work for decades trying to pinpoint and describe both the distinguishing characteristics of lesbian genitals and the 'effects' of lesbian sexual activity on women's sex organs.
2. For more detail on these findings see P. Townsend, N. Davidson and M. Whitehead, *Inequalities in Health* (Harmondsworth: Penguin, 1988).
3. Some research has suggested that lesbians are more likely than non-lesbian women to be in well-paid professional jobs, simply because not having to deal with the implications of heterosexuality (the problem of being better paid or in a more important job than your male partner, the question of seeing work as simply 'marking time' until marriage, the need to interrupt your career path to have children) leaves lesbians more free to take interesting work. This is discussed, for example, by Gill Dunne in her chapter 'Difference at Work:

Perceptions of Work from a Non-heterosexual Perspective' in Jackie Stacey, Ann Phoenix and Hilary Hinds (eds), *Working Out: New Directions for Women's Studies* (London: Taylor and Francis,1992). However, this applies only to a minority of women. In general lesbians earn women's wages (i.e., less than men!), are more likely to be single parents and are more likely to stay in low-paid, low-status work because of lack of job security and the risks of being sacked just for being lesbian.

4. For more on the prejudice of health care professionals, see Chapter 9.
5. For more on these ideas see Joan Cadden, *Meanings of Sex Difference in the Middle Ages* (Cambridge: Cambridge University Press, 1993) or Thomas Lacqueur, *Making Sex: Body and Gender from the Greeks to Freud* (New York: Harvard University Press, 1990).
6. All taken from George Henry, *Sex Variants: A Study of Homosexual Patterns* (London: Cassell and Company, 1950), pp. 1102, 1119, 1127.
7. Both doctors are cited in Michele Aina Barale's essay 'Below the Belt: (Un)covering the Well of Loneliness' in Diana Fuss (ed.), *Inside/Out: Lesbian Theories, Gay Theories* (London: Routledge,1991).
8. All summarized in Michael Ruse, *Homosexuality: a Philosophical Inquiry* (Oxford: Basil Blackwell, 1988).
9. Ricky Boden, 'Countertransference Response to Lesbians with Physical Disabilities and Chronic Illnesses' in Michael Shernoff and William Scott (eds), *The Sourcebook on Lesbian/Gay Health Care*, (Washington DC: National Lesbian and Gay Health Foundation, 1988, 2nd edn), p. 120.
10. Anyone interested in learning more is recommended to have a look at the chapter

'Orthodoxy within Disobedience: Lesbians and Feminists' in Tamsin Wilton, *Lesbian Studies: Setting an Agenda* (London: Routledge, 1995). Or, for a first-hand account from lesbians who were involved at the time, Sydney Abbott and Barbara Love, *Sappho was a Right-on Woman: A Liberated View of Lesbianism* (New York: Stein and Day, 1985).

11. C. Hepburn and B. Gutierrez, *Alive and Well: A Lesbian Health Guide* (Freedom, California: Crossing Press, 1994), p. 147.

12. Karen Kerner, 'Health Care Issues' in Karla Jay (ed.), *Dyke Life: From Growing Up to Growing Old, a Celebration of the Lesbian Experience* (London: Pandora, 1995).

13. Hepburn and Gutierrez are unambiguous in telling their readers, 'Don't drink milk' (note 11, p. 36).

14. Yes, it's all true, doctors really did say such things, and people really did believe them.

15. Dar, speaking in 'Fat Oppression Roundtable', in Regan McClure and Anne Vespry, *Lesbian Health Guide* (Toronto: Queer Press, 1994), p. 13.

16. See, for example, Lesley Doyal, *What Makes Women Sick: Gender and the Political Economy of Health* (London: Macmillan, 1995), Joan Busfield, *Men, Women and Madness: Understanding Gender and Mental Disorder* (London: Macmillan, 1996) or Jane Ussher, *Women's Madness: Misogyny or Mental Illness?* (London: Harvester Wheatsheaf, 1991).

Notes to Chapter 2

1. When I say 'smelly, sweaty men', I am referring to heterosexual men. Research done recently in Britain (Wilton 1996) suggests that women who use mixed gyms are all put off by three factors associated with the presence of men: the smell, the wet patches of sweat left on the equipment, and men's inconsiderate use of space and exercise equipment. Having exercised in gyms with a high proportion of gay men, I would suggest that the risk here is of asphyxiation by the fumes of expensive aftershave!

2. This 1946 WHO definition may be found in Peter Aggleton, *Health* (London: Routledge, 1990).

3. Sheridan Burton and Leonora Kane, 'Stress and Us' in Melba Wilson (ed.), *Healthy and Wise: The Essential Health Handbook for Black Women* (London: Virago, 1994), p. 32.

4. For a discussion of the health risks of coffee see Marjorie Ingall, 'Caffeine: The (Mostly) Good News', *Ms*, vol. vi, no. 2, September/October 1995, pp. 26–8.

5. Anne, another speaker at the lesbian fat oppression workshop.

6. I should mention here that, having been very overweight for twelve years, I lost around five stone by fairly simple changes in my eating habits (not by counting calories or following any formal diets but by cutting out chocolate and reducing the amount of food I ate). It wasn't a miracle cure for all my ills – my high blood pressure remained high – but it did make a dramatic improvement in my general health and wellbeing (my feet stopped hurting, I could run again, problems with my knee joints greatly improved) and the world became a much friendlier place. To my surprise, I also felt the loss of my fat self as quite painful. So I have personal experience of life as a fat lesbian, of the transformations which weight loss can bring and of the contradictory emotions which both may give rise to. Additionally, my being so fat was partly a survival strategy made necessary by a six-year relationship with a bulimic/anorexic woman. This personal experience inevitably shapes my thinking on the whole issue of weight and body image.

7. Carla Rice, 'Through Another Eye: Learning to Love Our Bodies and Ourselves' in R. McClure and A. Vespry (eds), *Lesbian Health Guide* (Toronto: Queer Press, 1994).

8. 'I define sadomasochism as any mode of behaviour that demonstrates hate and blocks the achievement of personal and political ambitions . . . Jolting the nerves of the body with pin pricks for sexual sensation is no better or worse than jolting the nerves of the body with caffeine for an alerting [*sic*] sensation' (Vivienne Walker-Crawford, 'The Saga of Sadie O. Massey' in Robin Ruth Linden *et al.* (eds), *Against Sadomasochism: A Radical Feminist Analysis* (San Francisco: Frog in the Well Press, 1982), p. 149).

9. Lesley Doyal, *What Makes Women Sick: Gender and the Political Economy of Health* (London: Macmillan, 1995).

10. See, for example, Joanne Hall, 'An Exploration of Lesbians' Recovery from Alcohol Problems' and Sharon Deevey and Lana Wall, 'How Do Lesbian Women Develop Serenity?', both in Phyllis Noerager Stern (ed.),

Lesbian Health: What Are the Issues?
(London: Taylor and Francis, 1993).

11. Sudden Infant Death Syndrome, sometimes called cot death. This refers to those babies who are found dead in their cots, apparently with no cause. It is clearly linked to smoking on the part of parents or carers.

12. The facts about coffee in this chapter are summarized from two papers: Sander Greenland, 'A Meta-analysis of Coffee Myocardial Infarction, and Coronary Death', *Epidemiology*, vol. 4 no. 4, July 1993, pp. 366–74, and Ichiro Kawachi, Graham Colditz and Catherine Stone, 'Does Coffee Drinking Increase the Risk of Coronary Heart Disease? Results from a Meta-analysis', *British Heart Journal*, no. 72, 1994, pp. 269–75. These two papers reach exactly opposite conclusions, which just goes to show . . . Thanks to George Davey Smith of Bristol University for bringing this research to my attention.

13. For more discussion of this, see Kathleen Erwin's paper 'Interpreting the Evidence: Competing Paradigms and the Emergence of Lesbian and Gay Suicide as a "Social Fact"', *International Journal of Health Services*, vol. 23, no. 3, 1993, pp. 437–53.

Notes to Chapter 4

1. Hunter and Polikoff cited in Ellen Lewin, 'Lesbianism and Motherhood: Implications for Child Custody' in Trudy Darty and Sandee Potter (eds), *Women-identified Women* (Palo Alto: Mayfield,1984). This quote is from a court case of 1976, but similar things continue to be reported in custody cases today.

2. This leads one to wonder *why* men need to reassure themselves that sexual pleasure is so unimportant to women. Of course, this has nothing to do with men's frequent failure to come up with the goods in between the sheets . . .

3. Anyone who is interested in finding out about the research findings which debunk all these myths is recommended to read Lisa Saffron's excellent book *Challenging Conceptions: Planning a Family by Self-insemination* (London: Cassell, 1994) or Diane Richardson's chapter 'Reproductive Technologies' in her book *Women, Motherhood and Childrearing* (London: Macmillan 1993).

4. Not much research has been done on this (surprise, surprise!). But it appears from what little has been done – for example in Ellen Lewin's work (note 1) – that lesbian mothers commonly tolerate grossly inadequate support from ex-husbands and male partners from fear of losing their children.

5. Susan Browne, Debra Connors and Nanci Stern (eds), *With the Power of Each Breath: A Disabled Women's Anthology* (San Francisco: Cleis Press, 1985), p. 274.

6. See Anne Finger, 'Claiming All of Our Bodies: Reproductive Rights and Disability' in Browne *et al.* (eds) (note 5).

7. See JoAnn leMaistre, 'Parenting' in Browne *et al.* (eds) (note 5).

8. See, for example, Margit Stange, 'The Broken Self: Fetal Alcohol Syndrome and Native American Selfhood' in Michael Ryan and Avery Gordon (eds), *Body Politics: Disease, Desire and the Family* (San Francisco: Westview Press, 1994).

9. Saffron (note 3) p. 1.

10. This may seem to be one disadvantage which lesbian parenting has compared to heterosexual parenting, but I have to say that I think the opposite is true! If more heterosexuals had to think through all the issues that lesbians confront in becoming parents, I suspect there would be fewer dysfunctional families. Being forced to think about so many additional variables makes us *better* prepared for the implications of parenting.

11. Although today's skilled needlewoman was yesterday's student, and they do have to learn, you are under no obligation to let them practise on your vagina.

12. See, for an especially spine-chilling example, the rant contributed by one 'Bev-Jo' to the popular collection *For Lesbians Only: A Separatist Anthology*, edited by Sarah Lucia-Hoagland and Julia Penelope (London: Onlywomen Press, 1988), in which she addresses 'Women who call themselves lesbians' (the implication being that *real* lesbians don't get pregnant) and spits that: 'Becoming a mother does mean . . . that [your] increased privilege will be at the expense of Lesbian non-mothers . . . that you are contributing to more hardship in all of our lives because your babies will be our future competition for housing, jobs, resources and possibly food and water . . . that *no matter what you do*, if you have a boy, he will terrorize and attack girls and, later, adult

women, and . . . it will not be a rare event if *you* are raped, beaten or killed by your son when he gets old enough' (pp. 315–17). Scary stuff!

13. Janet Kenney and Donna Tash, 'Lesbian Childbearing Couples' Dilemmas and Decisions' in Phyllis Noerager Stern (ed.), *Lesbian Health: What are the Issues?* (London: Taylor and Francis, 1993).
14. Research cited in Kenney and Tash, p. 123.
15. Kenney and Tash (note 13) p. 127.
16. Diane Richardson, *Women, Motherhood and Childrearing* (London: Macmillan, 1993), p. 81.

Notes to Chapter 5

1. These figures from Siobhan Hair (ed.), *Glasgow's Health: Women Count*, (Glasgow: Glasgow Healthy City Project, 1992).
2. Taken from Bristol Women's Studies Group (eds), *Half the Sky: An Introduction to Women's Studies* (London: Virago, 1979).
3. See, for example, Thomas Szasz, *The Myth of Mental Illness* (London: Secker and Warburg, 1961) or R. D. Laing, *The Politics of Experience and The Bird of Paradise* (Harmondsworth: Penguin, 1967).
4. The research carried out by Karen Armitage in 1971, which documented this discrimination in diagnostic practices, is widely reported. For a concise summary see Peter Aggleton, *Health* (London: Routledge,1990), pp. 127–8.
5. This is discussed in Susan Penfold and Gillian Walker's classic text *Women and the Psychiatric Paradox* (London: Eden Press,1983), pp. 96–7.
6. Lesley Doyal discusses this at length in her book *What Makes Women Sick: Gender and the Political Economy of Health* (London: Macmillan, 1995).
7. For more detailed discussion of these issues see Joan Busfield, *Men, Women and Madness: Understanding Gender and Mental Disorder* (London: Macmillan, 1996) or Jane Ussher, *Women's Madness: Misogyny or Mental Illness?* (London: Harvester Wheatsheaf, 1991).
8. In Doyal (note 6).
9. See Doyal (note 6).
10. Here is a selection of books which contain this material: Ussher (note 7), Busfield (note 7), Penfold and Walker (note 5), and Lesley

Doyal (note 6), plus Shere Hite, *The Hite Report: A Nationwide Study on Female Sexuality* (London: Macdonald, 1977), Luise Eichenbaum and Suzie Orbach, *What Do Women Want?* (London: Fontana, 1983), Phyllis Chessler, *Women and Madness* (New York: Doubleday, 1972) and Elaine Showalter, *The Female Malady: Women, Madness and English Culture 1830–1980* (London: Virago, 1987).
11. Ussher (note 7), p. 78.
12. This research is described in Sydney Abbott and Barbara Love, *Sappho was a Right-on Woman: A Liberated View of Lesbianism* (New York: Stein and Day, 1972) and Jeffrey Weeks, *Sexuality and its Discontents: Meanings, Myths and Modern Sexualities* (London: Routledge and Kegan Paul, 1985), and many other places.
13. Richard Isay, *Being Homosexual: Gay Men and Their Development* (Harmondsworth: Penguin, 1989). A point of clarification may be useful here. Psychiatrists belong to a branch of clinical medicine and have traditionally seen mental illness as organic in origin. They make use of treatments which affect the brain directly, such as drugs or electro-convulsive therapy (ECT), although they are becoming more open to less biological ideas. Psychoanalysts may operate within or outside of the clinical setting, but their ideas developed from the work of Sigmund Freud, who suggested that psychological problems in adult life stem from childhood experiences. Psychoanalysts use 'talking cures' rather than drugs to unearth the buried memories of events that gave rise to later symptoms of illness.
14. John Gonsiorek, 'Current and Future Developments in Gay/Lesbian Affirmative Mental Health Practice' in Michael Shernoff and William Scott (eds), *The Sourcebook on Lesbian and Gay Healthcare* (Washington DC: National Lesbian and Gay Health Foundation, 1988, 2nd edn), p. 108.
15. Discussed by Catherine Andrews and Jan Sherlock in their pamphlet *Women and Mental Health: Good Practices in Services for Lesbians and Bisexual Women* (London: Good Practices in Mental Health, 1994).
16. Jeffrey Weeks, *Coming Out: Homosexual Politics in Britain from the Nineteenth Century to the Present* (London: Quartet, 1990, rev.), p. 30.
17. Abbott and Love (note 12), p. 19.
18. Abbott and Love (note 12), p. 212.

19. I am not alone in my suspicion of the idea of 'lesbian merger'. For example, John Gonsiorek comments that it has altogether too much in common with 'psychoanalytic descriptions in the 1950s of the "pathology" of lesbianism' (Gonsiorek (note 14), p. 108). Yet open any book on lesbian psychology, lesbian health or lesbian social services, and nine times out of ten you will find the statutory article on merger in lesbian relationships. Such articles, it must be stressed, are based on completely inadequate research. But once they get published, they themselves become 'evidence' that this 'lesbian problem' exists.

20. Jane Futcher, 'Outlaws and Addicts: Lesbians and the Recovery Movement' in Karla Jay (ed.), *Dyke Life: From Growing Up to Growing Old, A Celebration of the Lesbian Experience* (London: Pandora, 1996), p. 342.

21. Sophie Laws, 'Women on the Verge', *Trouble and Strife*, no. 20, Spring 1991, pp. 8–12.

22. Gonsiorek (note 14).

23. Taken from the National Lesbian and Gay Survey's book *What a Lesbian Looks Like: Writings by Lesbians on Their Lives and Lifestyles* (London: Routledge, 1992), p. 101. I should add that I count myself among those lesbians whose history of 'clinical depression' ended with a transition from heterosexuality to lesbianism. That doesn't mean that I think being a lesbian 'cured' me, just that a different set of emotional resources became available to me. This is not something from which we can yet generalize.

24. I know what I'm talking about. Years of incapacitating panic attacks ceased magically when I gave up coffee. I'm a coffee fetishist – hand-grinding my favourite variety of fresh bean and using one of nine preferred ways of making the stuff – but I now try to stick resolutely to one cup a day.

25. See Doyal (note 6) for a discussion of this.

26. For more discussion of this, see Lois Arnold's report *Women and Self-injury* (Bristol: Bristol Crisis Service for Women, 1995).

27. Interviewed for Housk Randall and Ted Polhemus's book *The Customized Body* (London: Serpent's Tail, 1996).

28. Anonymous lesbian interviewed by Bristol Crisis Service for Women in their booklet *Women and Self-injury: For Friends and Family* (Bristol: Bristol Crisis Service for Women,1994), p. 14.

29. Bristol Crisis Service for Women, *Self-Help for Self-injury* (Bristol: Bristol Crisis Service for Women, 1994), p. 11.

30. In National Lesbian and Gay Survey (note 23), p. 99.

31. In National Lesbian and Gay Survey (note 23), p. 100.

32. Busfield (note 7), p. 234.

Notes to Chapter 6

1. From plenary presentation 'What are the needs of South Asian lesbians and gay men in terms of physical and mental health?', given at the *Health of the Lesbian, Gay and Bisexual Nation* Conference at Plymouth University, 16–17 March 1996.

2. Quoted in Jean Shapiro, *Ourselves Growing Older: Women Ageing with Knowledge and Power*, British edition (London: Fontana, 1988), p. 74.

3. Sharon Raphael and Mina Meyer, 'The Old Lesbian: Some Observations Ten Years Later' in Michael Shernoff and William Scott (eds), *The Sourcebook on Lesbian and Gay Health Care*, (Washington DC: National Lesbian and Gay Health Foundation, 2nd edn, 1988).

4. Both research findings from the Victorian Health Promotion Foundation Newsletter *Vic Health Letter* (special issue on older people), no. 5, August 1996, Melbourne, Australia.

5. For more on this see Lesley Doyal, *What Makes Women Sick: Gender and the Political Economy of Health* (London: Macmillan, 1995).

6. Shapiro (note 2), p. 1.

7. See, for example, Gill Dunne, 'Difference at Work: Perceptions of Work from a Non-heterosexual Perspective' in Jackie Stacey, Ann Phoenix and Hilary Hinds (eds), *Working Out: New Directions for Women's Studies* (London: Taylor and Francis, 1992).

8. Ellen Cole, 'Lesbian sexuality at Menopause', *Women's Global Network for Reproductive Rights Newsletter*, no. 42, January–March 1993, p. 37.

9. Lee Lynch, 'Forward' in *Off the Rag: Lesbians Writing on Menopause*, a book she edited with Akia Woods (Norwich, Vermont: New Victoria, 1996), p. 2.

10. For a discussion of this, see Marny Hall, 'Lesbian "Sex"' in Judith Barrington (ed.), *An Intimate Wilderness: Lesbian Writers on Sexuality* (Portland, Oregon: The Eighth Mountain Press, 1991).

11. Figures from Shapiro (note 2), p. 195.

12. Merrill Mushroom, 'My Life as a Volcano' in Lynch and Woods (note 9), p. 134.
13. From Shapiro (note 2), p. 195.
14. Dilation and curettage is a diagnostic technique which involves gently dilating the opening to the cervix so that a sample of tissue may be taken from the inside of the womb. It is also used to treat some conditions, for example by cutting away fibroids. It is a fairly routine procedure but if you are offered one, you can find out about the pros and cons by consulting *The New Our Bodies, Ourselves*.
15. Suspicious maybe, but I'm not the only one! For example, read the section on HRT in Shapiro (note 2) for a discussion of this interesting coincidence.
16. In the USA dental schools may offer a cheap alternative. For a booklet which gives details of cheap dental care options, send $1 to: Shipping Center Department DB31, Free and Low Cost Dental Care, PO Box 462, Elmira, NY 14902-0462. In Britain a few dentists are still offering treatment through the National Health Service, and some treatment may be available at dental hospitals. When chosing a dentist, check that s/he offers NHS treatment. Most private dentists offer reductions for pensioners, pregnant women and children, who all receive free treatment under the NHS.
17. In Shapiro (note 2).
18. See, for example, E. Cole and E. Rothblum, 'Lesbian Sex at Menopause: As Good as or Better than Ever' in B. Sang *et al.* (eds), *Lesbians at Midlife: The Creative Transition* (San Francisco: Spinsters, 1991).
19. In Shapiro (note 2).
20. See, for example, Barbara Macdonald with Cynthia Rich, *Look Me in the Eye: Old Women, Aging and Ageism* (London: The Women's Press, 1994) or Suzanne Neild and Rosalind Pearson, *Women Like Us* (London: Women's Press, 1992).
21. See, for example, articles in Regan McClure and Anne Vespry (eds), *Lesbian Health Guide* (Toronto: Queer Press, 1994).

Notes to Chapter 7

1. ME (myalgic encepahalomyelitis), sometimes called chronic fatigue syndrome, post-viral fatigue syndrome or Chronic Fatigue Immune Dysfunction Syndrom (CFIDS). For more

discussion of ME and lesbians, see the second half of this chapter.
2. Susan Lonsdale, *Women and Disability: The Experience of Physical Disability Among Women* (London: Macmillan, 1990), p. 142.
3. There is growing anecdotal evidence among lesbian communities in the USA, and certainly on a word-of-mouth basis among some lesbians in Britain, that chronic fatigue syndrome (sometimes, but not always, related to ME) appears to be strangely prevalent among lesbians. There is also a lively debate as to whether or not lesbians are more vulnerable to breast cancer than non-lesbian women. However, neither of these suggestions carries enough weight for us to regard lesbians as a 'risk group' for these or any other conditions.
4. Agnes Miles, *Women, Health and Medicine* (Milton Keynes: Open University Press, 1991), p. 111. Miles does not at any point recognize that the pressures she describes as affecting disabled *women* may be different for disabled *lesbians*, and that most of them represent the problem of heterosexuality, *not* the problem of disability!
5. Emily Levy, 'How the Rhino Got its Flaky Skin' in Susan Browne, Debra Connors and Nanci Stern (eds), *With the Power of Each Breath: A Disabled Women's Anthology* (San Francisco: Cleis Press, 1985), p. 35.
6. Sarah Pearlman, 'The Saga of Continuing Clash in Lesbian Community, or Will an Army of Ex-lovers Fail?' in *Lesbian Psychologies: Explorations and Challenges*, edited by the Boston Lesbian Psychologies Collective (Chicago: University of Illinois Press, 1987), p. 313.
7. Stephanie Sugars, 'Journal Piece' in Browne *et al.* (note 5), pp. 264–5.
8. Lonsdale (note 2), p. 47.
9. Lonsdale (note 2), p. 7.
10. Lonsdale (note 2), p. 71.
11. Rene Ungerecht, 'Age and Image' in Browne *et al.* (note 5). As an 'eleven-year-old quad', Ungerecht has been quadriplegic (without the use of both arrns and legs) for eleven years after a car accident when she was fifteen.
12. I speak from experience. During my heterosexual years I thought half an hour was a long time to spend making love. Becoming a lesbian changed all that, but getting ME changed it yet again and sex became a very tranquil, long-drawn-out business. Sometimes that can be wonderful, but it is

nice to have the choice, and when you are ill that choice is taken away.

13. Sophie, 'RSI – Taking the Strain', *Quim*, no. 3, Winter 1991, p. 42.

14. Lonsdale (note 2), p. 8.

15. This finding is reported in H. Lightfoot-Klein, 'The Sexual Experience and Marital Adjustment of Genitally Circumcized and Infibulated Females in the Sudan', *Journal of Sex Research*, no. 26, pp. 375–92.

16. Morag Christie, 'Hypocritical Oafs: ME', *Quim*, no. 4, 1992, p. 50.

Notes to Chapter 8

1. Jeffrey Weeks, *Invented Moralities: Sexual Values in an Age of Uncertainty* (Cambridge: Polity Press, 1995), p. 160.

2. Suniti Namjoshi and Gillian Hanscombe, *Flesh and Paper* (Seaton: Jezebel,1986).

3. Weeks (note 1), p. 161.

4. Weeks (note 1), p. 160.

5. Diane Silver, 'I Claim the Title of Widow', *Ms*, September/October 1995, p. 96.

6. Elizabeth Stuart, *Daring to Speak Love's Name: A Gay and Lesbian Prayer Book* (London: Hamish Hamilton, 1992), pp.128–9.

7. Silver (note 5), p. 96.

8. A. Powell Davies in Elizabeth Stuart (note 6), p. 141.

9. Stuart (note 6), p. 130.

10. This advice comes in Christopher Lukas and Henry M. Seiden's book *Silent Grief: Living in the Wake of Suicide* (London: Macmillan, 1987) p. 143, but it applies to everyone struggling to come to terms with the death of a partner or close friend.

11. Simon Watney, 'These Waves of Dying Friends: Gay Men, AIDS and Multiple Loss' in Peter Horne and Reina Lewis (eds), *Outlooks: Lesbian and Gay Sexualities and Visual Cultures* (London: Routledge, 1996) p. 166.

12. Lukas and Seiden (note 10), p. 71.

13. Lukas and Seiden (note 10), p. 71.

14. Lukas and Seiden (note 10), p. 143.

Notes to Chapter 9

1. See Lesley Doyal, *What Makes Women Sick: Gender and the Political Economy of Health* (London: Macmillan, 1995); Evelyn C. White (ed.), *The Black Women's Health Book: Speaking for Ourselves* (Seattle: Seal Press 1990) and Susan Browne, Debra Connors and Nanci Stern (eds), *With the Power of Each Breath: A Disabled Women's Anthology*, (San Francisco: Cleis Press, 1985).

2. For example, both *The Black Women's Health Book* and *With the Power of Each Breath* tokenize lesbians, and it has been a matter of bitter struggle to get lesbian issues on to the 'lesbian and gay' health care agenda.

3. Audre Lorde, 'Living with Cancer' in *The Black Women's Health Book* (note 1), p. 29.

4. Changes which are themselves no doubt related to the social and cultural impact of HIV, as well as to the post-Stonewall lesbian and gay political movements in Europe, North America and Australasia.

5. Cited in Regan McClure and Anne Vespry (eds), *Lesbian Health Guide* (Toronto: Queer Press, 1994), p. 237.

6. Cited in Susan Hemmings, 'Overdose of Doctors', published in *Spare Rib* in January 1986 and reprinted in Sue O'Sullivan (ed.), *Women's Health: A Spare Rib Reader* (London: Pandora, 1987), p. 131.

7. Liz Sayce, *Breaking the Link between Homosexuality and Mental Illness* (London: MIND, Celia Kitzinger, 1995); 'Heterosexism in Psychology', *The Psychologist*, September, 1990, pp. 391–2.

8. Hilary Graham, *Hardship and Health in Women's Lives* (London: Harvester Wheatsheaf, 1993), p. 6; Sue V. Rosser, 'Ignored, Overlooked or Subsumed: Research on Lesbian Health and Health Care', *National Women's Studies Association Journal*, vol. 5, no. 2, Summer 1993, pp.183–203.

9. LesBeWell volunteer, 'Lesbophobia in Nursing: A Case to Answer', *Dykenosis* (LesBeWell Newsletter), no. 2, p. 3.

10. Patricia Stevens, 'Lesbians' Health-related Experiences of Care and Non-care', *Western Journal of Nursing Research*, vol. 16, no. 6, 1994, pp. 639–59; Michigan Organization for Human Rights, *The Michigan Lesbian Health Survey*, MOHR Special Report, August 1991.

11. Michele Eliason, Carol Donelan and Carla Randall, 'Lesbian Stereotypes' in Phyllis Noerager Stern (ed.), *Lesbian Health: What are the Issues?* (London: Taylor and Francis, 1993), p. 46.

12. Judi Stein, 'Women's Community Health' in Ginny Vida (ed.), *Our Right to Love: A*

Lesbian Resource Book (Englewood Cliffs: Prentice-Hall, 1978), p. 117.

13. Stein (note 12).
14. Patricia Stevens, 'Lesbian Health Care Research: A Review of the Literature from 1970 to 1990' in Noergaer Stern (note 11), p. 20.
15. Grindl Dockery and Janet Price, *Final Report of the Research on the Sexual Health Needs of Lesbians, Bisexual Women and Women who have Sex with Women in Merseyside/Cheshire* (Liverpool: SHADY, 1996) and *Michigan Lesbian Health Survey* (note 10).
16. Stevens (note 14).
17. Stevens (note 14), Dockery and Price (note 15) and *Michigan Lesbian Health Survey* (note 10).
18. See, for example, Agnes Miles, *Women, Health and Medicine* (Buckingham: Open University Press, 1991) or Peggy Foster, *Women and the Health Care Industry: An Unhealthy Relationship?* (Buckingham: Open University Press, 1995).
19. If you choose to use them for safer sex, these latex gloves may already be familiar to you. If not, you can buy them in boxes of ten or more from pharmacists, drug stores or major supermarkets (where they are sold as lightweight gloves for household chores). You may like to be aware that if you incorporate latex gloves into your sex play and eroticize them, it can feel very odd when they are suddenly introduced into a health care examination!
20. Susan Trippet and Joyce Bain, 'Reasons American Lesbians Fail to Seek Traditional [*sic*] Health Care' in Noerager Stern (note 11). This survey used a sample of 503 lesbians, which is a reasonable sample size. However, the sample was recruited at three women's cultural events, so it is likely that there would be a bias in favour of alternative health care in such surroundings. A sample recruited at a women in management conference, for example, might be expected to give very different results!
21. See, for example, Eliason, Donelan and Randall (note 11), an account of research carried out with 278 nursing students.
22. See Stevens (note 14).
23. See, for example, Nicky Hart, *The Sociology of Health and Medicine* (Ormskirk: Causeway Books, 1985), which explains this very clearly.
24. If they're not, they should be! Get in there and wake them up.

Bibliography

Abbott, S. and Love, B. *Sappho was a Right-on Woman: A Liberated View of Lesbianism.* New York: Stein and Day, 1985.

Aggleton, P. *Health.* London: Routledge, 1990.

Ainley, R. *Death of a Mother: Daughters' Stories.* London: Pandora, 1991.

Alpert, H. (ed.) *We Are Everywhere: Writings by and about Lesbian Parents.* Boston: Crossing Press, 1988.

Andrews, C. and Sherlock, J. *Women and Mental Health: Good Practices in Service for Lesbians and Bisexual Women.* London: Good Practices in Mental Health, 1994.

Arnold, L. *Women and Self-injury: A Survey of 76 Women.* Bristol: Bristol Crisis Service for Women, 1995.

Arnup, K. *Lesbian Parenting: Living with Pride and Prejudice.* San Francisco: Gynergy Books, 1995.

Barale, M. A. 'Below the Belt: (Un)covering the Well of Loneliness' in D. Fuss (ed.), *Inside/Out: Lesbian Theories, Gay Theories.* London: Routledge, 1991.

Barrington, J. (ed.), *An Intimate Wilderness: Lesbian Writers on Sexuality.* Portland, Oregon: The Eighth Mountain Press, 1991.

Boden, R. 'Countertransference Response to Lesbians with Physical Disabilities and Chronic Illnesses' in M. Shernoff and W. Scott (eds), *The Sourcebook on Lesbian/Gay Health Care.* Washington DC: National Lesbian and Gay Health Foundation, 1988.

Boston, S. *Too Deep for Tears: Eighteen Years After the Death of My Son, Will.* London: Pandora, 1993.

Boston Lesbian Psychologies Collective (eds), *Lesbian Psychologies: Explorations and Challenges.* London: University of Illinois Press, 1987.

Boston Women's Health Book Collective (eds), *The New Our Bodies Ourselves: A Health Book By and For Women.* Harmondsworth: Penguin, 1989 (British edition edited by Angela Phillips and Jill Rakusen).

Bristol Crisis Service for Women. *Understanding Self Injury.* Bristol: Bristol Crisis Service for Women, 1994.

— *Self-help for Self-injury: A Guide for Women Struggling with Self-injury.* Bristol: Bristol Crisis Service for Women, 1994.

— *For Friends and Family: A Guide for Supporters of Women and Girls who Self-injure.* Bristol: Bristol Crisis Service for Women, 1994.

Bristol Women's Studies Group (eds), *Half the Sky: An Introduction to Women's Studies.* London: Virago, 1979.

Browne, S., Connors, D. and Stern, N. (eds), *With the Power of Each Breath: A Disabled Women's Anthology.* San Francisco: Cleis Press, 1985.

Burstow, B. *Radical Feminist Therapy*, London: Sage, 1992.

Busfield, J. *Men, Women and Madness: Understanding Gender and Mental Disorder.* London: Macmillan, 1996.

Cadden, J. *Meanings of Sex Difference in the Middle Ages.* Cambridge: Cambridge University Press, 1993.

Califia, P. *Sapphistry: The Book of Lesbian Sexuality.* Tallahassee: Naiad, 1988.

— *The Lesbian S/M Safety Manual.* Boston: Lace Publications/Alyson, 1988.

— *The Advocate Adviser.* Boston: Alyson, 1991.

Chessler, P. *Women and Madness.* New York: Doubleday, 1972.

Christie, M. 'Hypocritical Oafs: ME', *Quim*, no. 4, 1992, p. 50.

Cole, E. 'Lesbian Sexuality at Menopause', *Women's Global Network for Reproductive Rights Newsletter*, no. 42, January–March 1993, p. 37.

— and Rothblum, E. 'Lesbian Sex at Menopause: As Good as or Better than Ever' in B. Sang, J. Warshow and A. Smith (eds), *Lesbians at Midlife: The Creative Transition*. San Francisco: Spinsters, 1991.

Curtis, S. and Fraser, R. *Natural Healing for Women: Caring for Yourself with Herbs, Homoeopathy and Essential Oils*. London: Pandora, 1995.

Davies D. (ed.), *Pink Therapy: A Therapist's Guide to Working with Lesbians and Gay Men*. Milton Keynes: Open University Press, 1996.

Dockery, G. and Price, J. *Final Report of the Research on the Sexual Health Needs of Lesbians, Bisexual Women and Women who have Sex with Women in Merseyside/Cheshire*. Liverpool: SHADY, April 1996.

Doyal, L. *What Makes Women Sick: Gender and the Political Economy of Health*. London: Macmillan, 1995.

Dunne, G. 'Difference at Work: Perceptions of Work from a Non-heterosexual Perspective' in J. Stacey, A. Phoenix and H. Hinds (eds), *Working Out: New Directions for Women's Studies*. London: Taylor and Francis, 1992.

Eichenbaum, L. and Orbach, S. *What Do Women Want?* London: Fontana, 1983.

Eliason, M., Donelan, C. and Randall, C. 'Lesbian Stereotypes' in P. Noerager Stern (ed.), *Lesbian Health: What are the Issues?* London: Taylor and Francis, 1993.

Erwin, C. 'Interpreting the Evidence: Competing Paradigms and the Emergence of Lesbian and Gay Suicide as a "Social Fact"', *International Journal of Health Services* vol. 23, no. 3, 1993, pp. 437–53.

Faulder, C. *Whose Body Is It? The Troubling Issue of Informed Consent*. London: Virago, 1985.

Foster, P. *Women and the Health Care Industry: An Unhealthy Relationship?* Buckingham: Open University Press, 1995.

Futcher, J. 'Outlaws and Addicts: Lesbians and the Recovery Movement' in K. Jay (ed.), *Dyke Life: From Growing Up to Growing Old, A Celebration of the Lesbian Experience*. London: Pandora, 1996.

Gillespie-Sells, K. and Ruebain, D. *Disability OUT*. London: Channel 4 Television, 1992.

Gonsiorek, J. 'Current and Future Developments in Gay/Lesbian Affirmative Mental Health Practice' in M. Shernoff and W. Scott (eds), *The Sourcebook on Lesbian and Gay Health Care*. Washington: National Lesbian and Gay Health Foundation Ltd, 1988 (2nd edn).

Good Practices in Mental Health, *Women and Mental Health: An Information Pack of Mental Health Services for Women in the United Kingdom*. London: Good Practices in Mental Health, 1994.

Graham, H. *Hardship and Health in Women's Lives*. London: Harvester Wheatsheaf, 1993.

Greenland, S. 'A Meta-analysis of Coffee, Myocardial Infarction and Coronary Death', *Epidemiology*, vol. 4, no. 4, July 1993, pp. 366–74.

Hair, S. (ed.), *Glasgow's Health: Women Count*. Glasgow: Glasgow Healthy City Project, 1992.

Hall, M. *The Lavender Couch: A Consumer's Guide to Psychotherapy for Lesbians and Gay Men*. Boston: Alyson, 1985.

—— 'Lesbian "Sex"' in J. Barrington (ed.), *An Intimate Wilderness: Lesbian Writers on Sexuality*. Portland, Oregon: The Eighth Mountain Press, 1991.

Hart, N. *The Sociology of Health and Medicine*. Ormskirk: Causeway Books, 1985.

Hearn, K. 'Oi! What About Us?' in B. Cant and S. Hemmings (eds), *Radical Records: Thirty Years of Lesbian and Gay History*. London: Routledge, 1988.

Helminiack, D. *What the Bible Really Says About Homosexuality*. San Francisco: Alamo Square Press, 1994.

Hemmings, S. 'Overdose of Doctors' in S. O'Sullivan (ed.), *Women's Health: A Spare Rib Reader*. London: Pandora, 1987.

Henry, G. *Sex Variants: A Study of Homosexual Patterns*. London: Cassell and Company, 1950.

Hepburn, C. and Gutierrez, B. *Alive and Well: A Lesbian Health Guide*. Freedom, California: Crossing Press, 1994.

Hite, S. *The Hite Report: A Nationwide Study on Female Sexuality*. London: Macdonald, 1977.

Ingall, M. 'Caffeine: The (Mostly) Good News', *Ms*, vol. vi, no. 2, September/October 1995, pp. 26–8.

Isay, R. *Being Homosexual: Gay Men and Their Development*. Harmondsworth: Penguin, 1989.

Jay, K. (ed.), *Dyke Life: From Growing Up to Growing Old, a Celebration of the Lesbian Experience*. London: Pandora, 1995.

Kawachi, I., Colditz, G. and Stone, C. 'Does Coffee Drinking Increase the Risk of Coronary Heart Disease? Results from a Meta-analysis', *British Heart Journal*, no. 72, 1994, pp. 269–75.

Kenney, J. and Tash, D. 'Lesbian Childbearing Couples' Dilemmas and Decisions' in P. Noerager Stern (ed.), *Lesbian Health: What*

Are the Issues? London: Taylor and Francis, 1993.

Kerner, K. 'Health Care Issues' in K. Jay (ed.), *Dyke Life: From Growing Up to Growing Old, a Celebration of the Lesbian Experience*. London: Pandora, 1995.

Kitzinger, C. 'Heterosexism in Psychology', *The Psychologist*, September 1990, pp. 391–2.

— and Perkins, R. *Changing Our Minds*. London: Onlywomen Press, 1993.

Kitzinger, S. *Woman's Experience of Sex*. London: Dorling Kindersley, 1983.

Lacqueur, T. *Making Sex: Body and Gender from the Greeks to Freud*. Cambridge, Mass.: Harvard University Press, 1990.

Laing, R. D. *The Politics of Experience and the Bird of Paradise*. Harmondsworth: Penguin, 1967.

Laws, S. 'Women on the Verge', *Trouble and Strife*, no. 20, Spring 1991, pp. 8–12.

Lessing, J. 'Sex and Disability' in J. Loulan, *Lesbian Sex*. San Francisco: Spinsters Ink, 1984.

Levy, E. 'How the Rhino Got its Flaky Skin' in S. Browne *et al.* (eds), *With the Power of Each Breath: A Disabled Women's Anthology*. San Francisco: Cleis Press, 1985.

Lewin, E. 'Lesbianism and Motherhood: Implications for Child Custody' in T. Darty and S. Potter (eds), *Women-identified Women*. Palo Alto: Mayfield, 1984.

Lightfoot-Klein, H. 'The Sexual Experience and Marital Adjustment of Genitally Circumcized and Infibulated Females in the Sudan', *Journal of Sex Research*, no. 26, pp. 375–92.

Lonsdale, S. *Women and Disability: The Experience of Physical Disability Among Women*. London: Macmillan, 1990.

Lorde, A. *The Cancer Journals*. London: Sheba, 1980.

Lucia-Hoagland, S. and Penelope, J. (eds), *For Lesbians Only: A Separatist Anthology*. London: Onlywomen Press, 1988.

Lukas, C. and Seiden, H. M. *Silent Grief: Living in the Wake of Suicide*. London: Macmillan, 1987.

Lynch, L. and Woods, A. (eds), *Off the Rag: Lesbians Writing on Menopause*. Norwich, Vermont: New Victoria, 1996.

McClure, R. and Vespry, A. (eds), *Lesbian Health Guide*. Toronto: Queer Press, 1994.

Macdonald, B. with Rich, C. *Look Me in the Eye: Old Women, Aging and Ageism*. London: Women's Press, 1984.

Martin, A. *The Guide to Lesbian and Gay Parenting*. London: Pandora, 1993.

Michigan Organization for Human Rights, *The Michigan Lesbian Health Survey*. MOHR Special Report, August 1991.

Miles, A. *Women, Health and Medicine*. Buckingham: Open University Press, 1991.

Millet, K. *The Loony-Bin Trip*. London: Virago, 1990.

Muir-Mackenzie, A. and Orme, K. (eds), *Health of the Lesbian, Gay and Bisexual Nation: 1996 Conference Official Report*. Plymouth: The Harbour Centre, 1996.

Mushroom, M. 'My Life as a Volcano' in L. Lynch and A. Woods (eds), *Off the Rag: Lesbians Writing on Menopause*. Norwich, Vermont: New Victoria, 1996.

Namjoshi, S. and Hanscombe, G. *Flesh and Paper*. Seaton: Jezebel, 1986.

National Lesbian and Gay Survey (eds), *What a Lesbian Looks Like: Writings by Lesbians on Their Lives and Lifestyles*. London: Routledge, 1992.

Neild, S. and Pearson, R. (eds), *Women Like Us*. London: Women's Press, 1992.

Nissim, R. *Natural Healing in Gynaecology: A Manual for Women*. London: Pandora, 1996.

Noerager Stern, P. (ed.), *Lesbian Health: What Are the Issues?* London: Taylor and Francis, 1993.

Oliver, M. *The Politics of Disablement*. London: Macmillan, 1990.

O'Sullivan, S. and Parmar, P. *Lesbians Talk (Safer) Sex*. London: Scarlet, 1992.

Patton, C. and Kelly, J. *Making It: A Woman's Guide to Sex in the Age of AIDS*. New York: Firebrand, 1987.

Pearlman, S. 'The Saga of Continuing Clash in Lesbian Communities, or Will an Army of Ex-lovers Fail?' in Boston Lesbian Psychologies Collective (eds), *Lesbian Psychologies: Explorations and Challenges*. London: University of Illinois Press, 1987.

Penfold, S. and Walker, G. *Women and the Psychiatric Paradox*. London: Eden Press, 1983.

Perkins, R., Nadirshaw, Z., Copperman, J. and Andrews, C. (eds), *Women in Context: Good Practice in Mental Health Services for Women*. London: GPMH, 1996.

Pollack, S. and Vaughan, J. (eds), *Politics of the Heart: A Lesbian Parenting Anthology*. New York: Firebrand, 1987.

Rafkin, L. (ed.), *Different Mothers: Sons and Daughters of Lesbians Talk about their Lives*. San Francisco: Cleis Press, 1990.

Randall, H. and Polhemus, T. *The Customized Body*. London: Serpent's Tail, 1996.

Raphael, S. and Meyer, M. 'The Old Lesbian: Some Observations Ten Years Later' in M. Shernoff and W. Scott (eds), *The Sourcebook on Lesbian/Gay Health Care*. Washington DC: National Lesbian and Gay Health Foundation, 1988 (2nd edn).

Rice, C. 'Through Another Eye: Learning to Love Our Bodies and Ourselves' in R. McClure and A. Vespry (eds), *Lesbian Health Guide*. Toronto: Queer Press, 1994.

Richardson, D. *Safer Sex: The Guide for Women Today*. London: Pandora, 1990.

— *Women, Motherhood and Childrearing*. London: Macmillan, 1993.

Rosser, S. 'Ignored, Overlooked or Subsumed: Research on Lesbian Health and Health Care', *National Women's Studies Association Journal*, vol. 5, no. 2, Summer 1993, pp. 183–203.

Ruse, M. *Homosexuality: A Philosophical Inquiry*. Oxford: Basil Blackwell, 1988.

Saffron, L. *Challenging Conceptions: Planning a Family by Self-insemination*. London: Cassell, 1994.

Sang, B., Warshow, J. and Smith, A. *Lesbians at Midlife: The Creative Transition*. San Francisco: Spinsters Ink, 1991.

Sayce, L. *Breaking the Link Between Homosexuality and Mental Illness*. London: MIND (Mental Health Foundation), 1995.

Shakespeare, T., Gillespie-Sells, K. and Davies, D. *The Sexual Politics of Disability*. London: Cassell, 1996.

Shapiro, J. *Ourselves, Growing Older: Women Ageing with Knowledge and Power*. London: Fontana, 1988 (US edition by Doress and Segal, with the Boston Women's Health Book Collective).

Shernof, M. and Scott, W. (eds), *The Sourcebook on Lesbian/Gay Health Care*. Washington DC: National Lesbian and Gay Health Foundation Ltd, 1988 (2nd edn).

Showalter, E. *The Female Malady: Women, Madness and English Culture 1830–1980*. London: Virago, 1987.

Silver, D. 'I Claim the Title of Widow', *Ms*, September/October 1995, p. 96.

Skinner, C. J. 'A Case-controlled Study of the Sexual Health Needs of Lesbians', *Genitourinary Medicine*, vol. 72, no. 4, 1996, pp. 277–80.

Smith, G. and Nairne, K. *Dealing with Depression*. London: Women's Press, 1995 (rev edn).

Sophie, 'RSI: Taking the Strain', *Quim*, no. 3, Winter 1991, p. 42.

Stacey, J., Phoenix, A. and Hinds, H. (eds), *Working Out: New Directions for Women's Studies*. London: Taylor and Francis, 1992.

Stange, M. 'The Broken Self: Fetal Alcohol Syndrome and Native American Selfhood' in M. Ryan and A. Gordon (eds), *Body Politics: Disease, Desire and the Family*. San Francisco: Westview Press, 1994.

Stein, J. 'Women's Community Health' in G. Vida (ed.), *Our Right to Love: A Lesbian Resource Book*. Englewood Cliffs: Prentice-Hall, 1978.

Stevens, P. 'Lesbian Health Care Research: A Review of the Literature from 1970 to 1990' in P. Noerager Stern (ed.), *Lesbian Health: What are the Issues?* London: Taylor and Francis, 1993.

— 'Lesbians' Health-related Experiences of Care and Non-care', *Western Journal of Nursing Research*, vol. 16, no. 6, 1994, pp. 639–59.

Stoppard, M. *Being a Well Woman: How to Achieve and Maintain Personal Fitness, Health and Happiness*. New York: Holt, Rinehart and Winston, 1982.

Stuart, E. *Daring to Speak Love's Name: A Gay and Lesbian Prayer Book*. London: Hamish Hamilton, 1992.

Sugars, S. 'Journal Piece' in D. Browne *et al.* (eds), *With the Power of Each Breath: A Disabled Women's Anthology*. San Francisco: Cleis Press, 1985.

Szasz, T. *The Myth of Mental Illness*. London: Secker and Warburg, 1961.

Taylor, D., Taylor, S. and Coverdale, A. (eds), *Women of the Fourteenth Moon: Writings on Menopause*. Boston: Crossing Press, 1991.

Townsend, P., Davidson, N. and Whitehead, M. *Inequalities in Health: The Black Report and the Health Divide*. Harmondsworth: Penguin, 1988.

Trippet, S. and Bain, J. 'Reasons American Lesbians Fail to Seek Traditional Health Care' in P. Noerager Stern (ed.), *Lesbian Health: What are the Issues?* London: Taylor and Francis 1993.

Ungerecht, R. 'Age and Image' in S. Browne *et al.* (eds), *With the Power of Each Breath: A Disabled Women's Anthology*. San Francisco: Cleis Press, 1985

Ussher, J. *Women's Madness: Misogyny or Mental Illness?* London: Harvester Wheatsheaf, 1991.

Walker-Crawford, V. 'The Saga of Sadie O. Massey' in R. Linden, D. Pagano, D. Russell and S. Star (eds), *Against Sadomasochism: A Radical Feminist Analysis*. San Francisco: Frog in the Well Press, 1982.

Watney, S. 'These Waves of Dying Friends: Gay Men, AIDS and Multiple Loss' in P. Horne and R. Lewis (eds), *Outlooks: Lesbian and Gay Sexualities and Visual Cultures*. London: Routledge, 1996.

Weeks, J. *Sexuality and its Discontents: Meanings, Myths and Modern Sexualities*. London: Routledge and Kegan Paul, 1985.

—— *Coming Out: Homosexual Politics in Britain from the Nineteenth Century to the Present*. London: Quartet, 1990 (rev. edn).

—— *Invented Moralities: Sexual Values in an Age of Uncertainty*. Cambridge: Polity Press, 1995.

Werthheimer, A. *A Special Scar: The Experiences of People Bereaved by Suicide*. London: Routledge, 1991.

White, E. C. (ed.), *The Black Women's Health Book: Speaking for Ourselves*. Seattle: Seal Press, 1990.

Wilson, M. (ed.), *Healthy and Wise: The Essential Health Handbook for Black Women*. London: Virago, 1994.

Wilton, T. *Lesbian Studies: Setting an Agenda*. London: Routledge, 1995.

—— 'A Healthy Performance? Queer Theory and Health Promotion', paper presented at the 1996 Annual Conference of the Medical Sociology Group of the British Sociological Association, Edinburgh University.

Woodham, A. *HEA Guide to Complementary Medicine and Therapies*. London: Health Education Authority, 1994.

Index